DIVINE ENERGY
The Ultimate Source of Human Healing

Dr. Scott A. Johnson

COPYRIGHT © 2025, by Scott A. Johnson

All Rights Reserved. No part of this publication may be reproduced or transmitted in any form or by any means, electronic or mechanical, including photocopying and recording, or introduced into any information storage and retrieval system without the written permission of the copyright owner. Brief quotations may be used in reviews prepared for magazines, blogs, newspapers, or broadcasts.

Divine Energy: The Ultimate Source of Human Healing / Scott A. Johnson

Cover design: Scott A. Johnson
Cover Copyright © 2025, by Scott A. Johnson

ISBN-13: 979-8988720652

Published by Scott A. Johnson Professional Writing Services, LLC: Orem, UT

Discover more books by Scott A. Johnson at authorscott.com/shop/

DISCLAIMERS OF WARRANTY AND LIMITATION OF LIABILITY

The author provides all information on an "as is" and "as available" basis and for informational purposes only. The author makes no representations or warranties of any kind, expressed or implied, as to the information, materials, or products mentioned. Every effort has been made to ensure accuracy and completeness of the information contained; however, it is not intended to replace any medical advice or to halt proper medical treatment, nor diagnose, treat, cure, or prevent any health condition or disease.

Always consult a qualified medical professional before using any dietary supplement or natural product, engaging in physical activity, or modifying your diet; and seek the advice of your physician with any questions you may have regarding any medical condition. Always consult your OB/GYN if you are pregnant or think you may become pregnant before using any dietary supplement or natural product, and to ensure you are healthy enough for exercise or any dietary modifications. The information contained in this book is for educational and informational purposes only, and it is not meant to replace medical advice, diagnosis, or treatment in any manner. Never delay or disregard professional medical advice. Use the information solely at your own risk; the author accepts no responsibility for the use thereof. This book is sold with the understanding that neither the author nor publisher shall be liable for any loss, injury, or harm allegedly arising from any information or suggestion in this book.

The Food and Drug Administration (FDA) has not evaluated the statements contained in this book. The information and materials are not meant to diagnose, prescribe, or treat any disease, condition, illness, or injury. You are encouraged to seek the most current information and medical care from your healthcare professional.

CONTENTS

Foreword 7

CHAPTER ONE: Humans Are Energetic beings 11

CHAPTER TWO: Divine Energy, Stress, Emotions, and Cellular Memory 33

CHAPTER THREE: The Body is the Divinely Designed Healer 47

CHAPTER FOUR: What is Divine Energy? 53

CHAPTER FIVE: The Divine Interconnectedness Between All Life 67

CHAPTER SIX: Lifestyle Behaviors that Harness Divine Energy: Nutrition, Physical Activity, and Relaxation Techniques 83

CHAPTER SEVEN: Channeling Divine Energy with Energy Healing Techniques 99

CHAPTER EIGHT: Connecting with Divine Energy Through Sound and Novel Technology 141

CHAPTER NINE: The Influence of Natural Solutions on Divine Energy: Essential Oils and Dietary Supplements 159

CHAPTER TEN: Harness Divine Energy and Be Healthy ... 175

References 185

Index 197

Foreword

As a man of deep faith, but also operating within the sciences, I often looked at energy healing modalities as "woo woo" and not grounded in evidence. Early in my career in natural health, my mind was too closed to even let this concept exist. However, as I continued to ponder on how God works and by what power or authority He heals us, I began to make a subtle connection between Him and energy, particularly in relation to His Light.

As a man of deep faith, grounded in the teachings of God, yet also committed to the rigors of science, I have long wrestled with reconciling these two worlds. I never questioned the existence of God, but I sincerely desired to connect Him and His workings to the sciences. I held a profound desire to acquire more wisdom and understanding of the laws by which He promotes healing within the human body so I could share it with others. The more I learned from science and how things like the human body operate, the more my awe for and belief in God increased.

My early days in natural health were marked by skepticism toward anything that seemed extremely fringe or ungrounded in hard evidence. Among these was the concept of energy healing—a practice I dismissed as unfounded and unscientific. My analytical mind had erected barriers that refused to even entertain the possibility of its existence, much less its validity.

But life has a way of challenging our preconceived notions, often in unexpected ways. As I delved deeper into my understanding of how God works and by what power or authority He creates, sustains, and restores (heals) all things, my perspective began to shift. Questions lingered: Since God is the Creator of all things, how does His power manifest in the physical world? Could His Light, often described in Scripture as a source of life and healing, be more than metaphorical?

Could it hold an energetic, measurable quality that connects faith and science?

The Bible often speaks of God as Light—"The Lord is my light and my salvation" (Psalm 27:1), "I am the light of the world: he that followeth me shall not walk in darkness, but shall have the light of life" (John 8:12), and "God is light; in Him, there is no darkness at all" (1 John 1:5). For centuries, theologians have interpreted this light as spiritual guidance and divine purity. Yet, as I reflected more deeply, I began to see another layer of meaning. Light, in the physical sense, is energy. It sustains life on Earth, enables vision, and serves as the foundation of biological and ecological systems. Could the Light of God, so central to spiritual teachings, also hold the key to understanding energy and healing on a scientific level?

Modern science has revealed that the human body is not merely flesh and bone; it is a dynamic, energetic system. From the electrical impulses of the heart and brain to the biophotons emitted by our cells, life is pulsating with energy. When I began to explore these concepts with an open mind and prayed for greater knowledge and wisdom, I realized that they aligned with the belief that we are "fearfully and wonderfully made" (Psalm 139:14). Our intricate design speaks not only to divine craftsmanship but also to the idea that energy might be the medium through which God interacts with His creations.

This realization profoundly impacted my journey. What if energy healing, often dismissed as pseudoscience, is a reflection of divine mechanisms we have yet to fully understand? What if it is another way that God's Light works within us, bringing harmony to our physical, emotional, mental, and spiritual selves? Just as prayer and faith can lead to healing that defies medical explanation, perhaps energy-based practices operate as extensions of God's Light, guided by His will and wisdom. And in his loving mercy, He empowers humans to channel His energy to the benefit of others.

In this book, I invite you to explore the intersection of faith, science, and energy with an open and critical mind. Together, we will examine how God's design of the universe and the human body reveals an incredible harmony of the physical and the spiritual. We will challenge outdated notions, embrace both evidence and mystery, and ultimately seek to understand how God's Light—a concept that transcends the confines of both theology and science—can illuminate the path to healing and wholeness.

This journey is not about replacing faith with science or vice versa. It is about discovering how the two can coexist and enrich each other, pointing us to the truth that God's ways are both awe-inspiring and profoundly practical. As you read, I encourage you to remain receptive—open to the idea that God's power and presence are not confined to the intangible but are woven into the very fabric of creation. Most importantly, receptive to the teachings of the Spirit, which is the source of all Truth. One of the roles of the Holy Ghost is to reveal and affirm the truth, and all honest seekers of the truth can feel His influence. His Light is in us, around us, and through us, bringing balance, healing, and the ultimate reminder of His love.

Let us step into that Light together.

Scott A. Johnson

CHAPTER ONE

Humans Are Energetic Beings

Human beings are fundamentally energetic beings, with every organelle, cell, organ, and system driven by intricate energy processes. This energy governs not only our physical functions but also our mental, emotional, and spiritual well-being. At the core of this concept lies the idea that health and healing are deeply rooted in maintaining the harmonious flow and balance of energy within and around the body. And, as this book proposes, this energy can be wielded by humans to promote miraculous healing.

The Energy of Life: Understanding the Interconnectedness of Emotions, Health, and Healing

On a cellular level, energy drives life processes through bioelectrical and biochemical pathways. Energy also connects to emotional and mental states, which significantly impact health. Emotions like joy and gratitude enhance energetic flow, promoting healing, while stress and negativity disrupt it, leading to disease. Practices such as meditation, breathwork, and prayer are known to restore energetic balance, aligning physical and emotional states with health.

While giving a lecture at the University of Pittsburgh in 1934, Albert Einstein stated, "We are dealing with fundamental problems of energy and matter, and the treatment of illness by energy is in principle conceivable." Furthermore, his vision of future medicine is consistent with a belief in the intimate relationship between electromagnetism and life. He boldly theorized that "Future medicine will be the medicine of frequencies." As usual, Einstein was ahead of his time in theorizing a fundamental core to healing—energy!

Likewise, Nikola Tesla, the genius inventor and visionary, believed that everything in the universe, including the human body, is made of energy. Ralph Bergstresser claims he heard Tesla famously proclaim, "If you want to find the secrets of the universe, think in terms of energy, frequency, and vibration." Tesla's insights and contributions to electricity and electromagnetism are now fueling innovation in the field of energy medicine.

Ultimately, embracing our energetic nature reminds us of the interconnectedness of mind, emotions, body, and spirit, illuminating the profound power of energy in achieving and sustaining optimal health. This model of human health and healing is supported by evidence extracted from sciences and theories entrenched in physics, bioenergetics, quantum biology, and modern techniques that measure the energy (electrical activity) in the body. While technical, this information is included to provide evidence using validated scientific methods to support our hypothesis that we are energetic beings. A less technical summary is included in dark gray and italics.

Physics: The Study of How the Universe Works

Physics is a fundamental science that seeks to understand the basic principles governing the natural world, including the nature of matter, energy, space, and time. In essence, it pursues knowledge and understanding that explains how the universe works, from the smallest known particles to the largest galaxies. To accomplish this, physics develops theoretical models—

classical mechanics, relativity, thermodynamics, quantum mechanics, electromagnetism, optics, and acoustics—that describe and predict phenomena. Findings in physics are used to solve practical problems in various fields, ranging from engineering to medicine. Modern technologies that leverage physics to enhance our daily lives include computers, smartphones, medical imaging devices, and solar panels.

While the concept of "body energy" isn't a direct physical quantity like mass or velocity, we can use various physical principles to indirectly measure its manifestations. Direct calorimetry measures the heat produced by the body. The body creates heat through metabolic activities, which involves the conversion of energy to heat. Direct calorimetry captures and measures this heat to calculate energy expenditure. Indirect calorimetry measures the amounts of oxygen consumed and carbon dioxide produced by the body, which estimates the body's metabolic rate—a measure of energy expenditure. Bioelectric impedance analysis measures body composition by calculating the resistance of a small electrical current traveling through the body. These are just a few examples of how physics permits quantifying energy in the body.

Physics is the study of how the universe works. It helps us understand things like light, sound, and how things move. Scientists use physics to measure how much energy our bodies contain using special tools. One way is to measure how much heat we give off. Another way is to measure how much oxygen we breathe in and carbon dioxide we breathe out. We can also use electricity to measure how much water and muscle we have, which helps us understand our energy levels.

Unlocking Life's Energy: The Science of Bioenergetics and Its Role in Cellular Function

Bioenergetics is a field of science that focuses on the flow of energy in biological systems. It investigates processes through which living organisms create, convert, and utilize energy to perform biological functions, including growth, reproduction, movement, and maintenance of cellular and bodily functions. From a foundational level, all cells function on the principles of bioenergetics because cells must produce, utilize, and regenerate ATP (adenosine triphosphate), or the "energy currency" of the cell, to function efficiently. Bioenergetics is also crucial to understanding how nutrition affects energy metabolism in humans, metabolic disorders such as diabetes, and exercise physiology. Overall, bioenergetics provides invaluable insights by bridging biology, chemistry, and physics, ultimately revealing how life sustains itself through energy management and transformation.

Bioenergetics is the study of how living things use energy. It's like the energy system of a cell. Cells need energy to grow, move, and repair themselves. This energy comes from food, which is broken down to make a special kind of energy called ATP. Understanding bioenergetics helps us learn about how our bodies work, how we get energy from food, and why sometimes our bodies don't work as they should, like in diseases such as diabetes.

Insights into Fundamental Processes that Govern Life and Health Through Quantum Biology

Quantum biology is an interdisciplinary field that applies principles from quantum mechanics to biological systems. It explores phenomena that occur at the molecular and cellular levels, where quantum mechanical effects can influence biological processes. While quantum biology is still a relatively novel field, it has been gaining attention for its potential implications for understanding complex biological phenomena and human health. By elucidating how quantum phenomena influence processes like metabolism, cellular signaling, and other biochemical reactions, we can gain deeper insights into how disturbances in these processes contribute to diseases. It can also better inform practitioners and users of healing solutions by improving our understanding of enzyme mechanisms or molecular interactions, leading to more effective and targeted treatments. Lastly, diseases like cancer, neurodegenerative disorders, and metabolic syndromes likely involve quantum effects at the cellular or molecular level. Understanding these effects may open promising avenues for research that could lead to new treatment strategies. As our understanding of quantum biology expands, it will provide valuable insights into the fundamental processes that govern life and health.

Quantum biology is a new kind of science that looks at how tiny things, like atoms, can affect living things. Scientists are learning that these tiny things can influence how our bodies work, from how we get energy to how our brains think. By understanding this, we might be able to find new ways to treat diseases and keep people healthy. It's like unlocking a secret code to life itself!

Illuminating the Body's Electrical Activity via Modern Imaging Techniques

Modern imaging techniques that measure electrical activity in the body are essential for understanding physiological processes, diagnosing diseases, and guiding treatments. Various methods have been developed to provide insights into electrical activity in the heart, brain, muscles, and other tissues.

Electroencephalography (EEG) measures electrical activity in the brain, allowing the diagnosis of seizure disorders, brain tumors, head and brain injuries, and the monitoring of brain activity, function, and behavior.

Electrocardiography (ECG or EKG) measures electrical activity of the heart, producing a waveform that provides information about heart rhythm, size of heart chambers, and the presence of any heart conditions.

Electromyography (EMG) is used to measure the electrical activity of muscles. It is a valuable tool to assess the health of both muscles and the nerve cells that control them and can be employed to diagnose neuromuscular disorders and monitor rehabilitation processes.

While primarily used for brain imaging, *Functional Magnetic Resonance Imaging (fMRI)* can also be used to infer electrical activity by detecting changes in blood flow and oxygenation, which correlate with neural activity. Used in this way, fMRI can help us understand brain connectivity.

Magnetoencephalography (MEG) measures the magnetic fields produced by electrical currents flowing in the brain. It is a complementary technique to EEG, with better spatial resolution, and useful for mapping brain function, studying cognitive processes, and determining brain regions involved in various functions.

Electrical Impedance Tomography (EIT) measures the electrical conductivity of tissues. It is used to monitor lung function, detect breast tumors, and assess other conditions where tissue conductivity changes.

All these techniques measure electrical activity in humans in real time and contribute to a deeper understanding of physiological processes. They are quantifiable evidence that humans are energetic beings. Indeed, physics and bioenergetics confirm that every cell in the human body generates electric currents, which produce measurable electromagnetic fields. Living cells emit low levels of light (biophotons), which are thought to play a role in cellular communication. These biophotons may even regulate biological processes and signal the body's state of health. We'll explore biophotons in greater detail in the next chapter.

It's actually quite ironic that energy medicine and healing modalities are almost exclusively found in complementary practices like acupuncture, qigong, kinesiology, and Reiki when modern science can measure energy in the form of electricity in the body. Each of these anciently practiced techniques is based on the concept of energy (e.g., "Qi" in Chinese medicine, "Ki" in Japanese medicine, "Prana" in Ayurveda) flowing through the body. Blockages or imbalances in this energy along energy pathways in the body are believed to be the root cause of illness.

Unlocking the Body's Electrical Signals as a Diagnostic Aid

In reality, many people are unknowingly measuring energy (electrical activity) in their bodies every single day by wearing a smartwatch or ring. One of the key technologies behind these devices is galvanic skin response (GSR), a phenomenon that occurs when electrical activity is measured in the body.

GSR devices measure the resistance or conductance of the skin, which changes in response to emotional arousal. When a person is stressed, excited, or experiencing emotional turmoil, their sweat glands become more active, leading to increased moisture on the skin's surface. This moisture decreases electrical resistance, making the skin more conductive. The data collected through GSR is then used to provide insights into an individual's stress levels, emotional states, and overall mental well-being.

Smartwatches and rings also utilize optical sensors based on photoplethysmography (PPG) technology. These sensors emit light (usually green LEDs) onto the skin and measure the amount of light that is reflected back. The pulsation of blood vessels as the heart beats causes the light reflected to change, allowing the device to calculate heart rate and other vital signs. Additionally, accelerometer data from movement patterns are combined with heart rate and other vital signs to estimate different sleep stages, including light, deep, and REM sleep. Some devices even directly measure heart rate variability (HRV), providing a more accurate picture of the autonomic nervous system's activity.

Other devices take a more comprehensive approach by combining electrical impedance analysis and photobiomodulation with bio-photonic analysis. These devices measure light transmission and impedance, analyzed using a complex algorithm to generate a report on various biomarkers. This report provides insights into the body's energetic and functional states, highlighting areas of balance and imbalance. Based on the analysis, recommendations are made for nutritional supplements, essential oils, herbs, or other natural products that may help improve the body's energetic and functional status.

By analyzing key biomarkers and providing targeted recommendations, these devices empower individuals to take a more active role in their health and wellness. Whether it's stress management, sleep improvement, or troubling conditions, these devices offer a unique perspective on the body's complex systems and provide a framework for making informed lifestyle choices.

As technology continues to evolve, devices that harness the power of electrical signals and bio-photonic analysis are poised to play a significant role in shaping the future of personalized health and wellness. By leveraging these innovative technologies, individuals can gain a deeper understanding of their bodies and make informed decisions to optimize their well-being.

The Placebo Effect: Revealing the Mind-Body-Spirit Connection

Even the placebo effect—healing through belief, expectations, and intention—demonstrates how body energy, most likely originating from the brain, can influence physical health. Neurobiological studies have identified changes in multiple pathways—dopaminergic, opioidergic, vasopressinergic, and endocannabinoidergic—as crucially involved in symptom relief and healing.[1] So, physiological changes, directed and powered by divine energy triggered by a placebo, are detectable via changes in neurotransmitters systems in the brain. It's like our thoughts trigger a cascade of energy-driven events that assemble and rally divine healing energy and then direct it to areas of the body for healing purposes.

The placebo effect is so powerful that even physicians leverage it as a treatment for their patients. A 2008 survey of nearly 700 internal medicine doctors and arthritis specialists published in the *British Medical Journal* found that about half admitted to prescribing placebos regularly—two to three times per month.[2] Further confirmation that doctors understand the mind-body connection comes from findings of the survey that of those prescribing placebos, only 5 percent informed their patients they were receiving a placebo. When even physicians are willing to prescribe "inert" substances (sugar pills or saline) or physiologically active agents (vitamins, OTC drugs, and antibiotics) not aimed at treating the patient's specific illness solely to promote positive expectation of healing, it's a powerful testimony for the ability of the mind to access the conduit of divine energy for healing.

The Nocebo Effect: How Beliefs Shape Health Outcomes

More evidence that belief in something producing an outcome, positive or negative, is the nocebo effect. The opposite of the placebo effect, the nocebo effect is a phenomenon where a person experiences negative symptoms or outcomes because of being told or believing that they will experience them. Like the placebo effect, the nocebo effect occurs due to psychological (conditioning and negative expectations) and neurobiological (role of cholecystokinin, endogenous opioids, and dopamine) mechanisms. A high percentage of side effects reported in the placebo arms of clinical trials supports the nocebo effect.

For example, a review of clinical trials and the side effects reported in placebo arms found that experiences of participants conclusively explain the occurrence of a placebo or nocebo effect.[3] One trial reported in the review noted participants receiving an anticonvulsant placebo experienced common side effects of an actual anticonvulsant—anorexia and memory difficulties. In other words, if a trial participant believes they will have a negative effect, they are highly likely to experience the exact adverse effect they believe will occur. The findings of this review bring attention to the important role that healthcare practitioners play in patient-clinician interactions.

Verbal and nonverbal communications from healthcare professionals convey messages that can lead to numerous unintentional negative consequences and a nocebo response. Simple phrasing of side-effect risks can avert or elicit a nocebo effect. For example, if the healthcare professional says, "Twelve percent of patients experience X side effect when taking this medication" as opposed to "The great majority of patients tolerate this medication very well," the patient has a higher risk of a nocebo effect.

Progressive Modern Practices that Rely on Energy Healing Techniques

While conventional medicine primarily focuses on biochemistry, research suggests that bioenergetics may complement physical healing. More recently, even progressive Western medical practices have relied on energy healing techniques. Pulsed Electromagnetic Field (PEMF) therapy, an evidence-based medical technology, uses electromagnetic fields to stimulate healing, particularly for bone fractures and chronic pain.[4,5] Similarly, brain stimulation—therapies that activate or inhibit the brain with electricity—is being explored as a treatment for depression.[6] Transcutaneous Electrical Nerve Stimulation (TENS) is a therapy that delivers electrical pulses to nerve endings through the skin to relieve pain.[7] These progressive treatments are dipping their toes into energy medicine, perhaps without the practitioners even knowing it.

Even more traditional Western medicine devices rely upon electricity or energy to maintain life. A pacemaker leverages electrical pulses to regulate the heartbeat, while a defibrillator shocks the heart with electricity to restore a normal heart rhythm. Electricity is a form of energy that comes from the flow of tiny particles called electrons. Movement of these electrons creates electrical energy, which can be harnessed for various purposes. Clearly, Western medicine trusts energy (electrical) therapies for diagnostics and healing even if its practitioners fail or refuse to recognize this fact.

Harnessing the Heart's Energy: Exploring the Biofield and Its Impact on Emotional and Physical Well-Being

Another indication of energy being a vital force in human health is the fact that humans—and other living organisms—each have a measurable biofield that is influenced by energetic systems.[8] A human biofield can be observed through different equipment and methods, including Kirlian photography, biofield imaging devices, and psychophysiological measurements. Kirlian photography is a technique that captures the visible aura around objects, including humans, based on high-frequency electrical discharge. While its interpretations are debatable and contentious, it is suggestive of a human bioenergetic field. Devices such as gas discharge visualization and other energy field measuring tools claim to capture the biofield. Critics argue that while these tools measure something, it may not accurately reflect a distinct biofield as traditionally conceptualized. Seeing isn't always believing! Lastly, heart rate variability (HRV)—more to come on this—and galvanic skin response are biological measures that infer how the body interacts with its environment. Although these are not direct measures of a biofield, they do measure changes in the life force, or divine energy, in the body. Dr. Konstantin Korotkov undertook a range of studies showing that therapies that influence energy, such as therapeutic touch, magnet therapy, hypnosis, and qigong, produce observable changes in energy emission patterns.[9] This discussion around biofields intersects with broader issues in mind-body connections and holistic health that warrant further exploration and validation.

Remarkably, the heart's electrical energy is roughly sixty times greater in amplitude than the electrical activity generated by the brain.[10] This suggests that the heart plays a greater role in harnessing divine energy than the brain, making the heart the center of human existence. This is why the heart (emotions) often triumphs over reason (the brain) because emotions are deeply tied to our survival, identity, and ability to connect with others.

The heart generates a complex electromagnetic field that extends beyond the physical body. The electromagnetic activity of the heart is influenced by various factors, including emotional states. When a person is in a state of genuine love or care, this electromagnetic field exhibits specific characteristics that indicate clarity or coherence.[11] The term "coherence" refers to a state where the heart's rhythms are smooth and ordered, as opposed to erratic or chaotic patterns. When a person experiences positive emotions such as love, compassion, or care, their heart rhythms tend to become more ordered and harmonious. This coherence in heart rhythms can lead to a clearer and more stable electromagnetic field, which researchers suggest may be associated with improved emotional and physical well-being. This connection between emotions and physiological responses underscores the holistic nature of health, where emotional well-being can significantly impact physical health.

Emerging evidence even suggests that we can share our heart energy with others through touch or close proximity.[12] A 20-second hug can be a surprisingly powerful form of healing due to several psychological and physiological benefits that arise from this simple act of physical affection.[13] Hugging stimulates the release of oxytocin, often referred to as the "love hormone" or "bonding hormone." Oxytocin promotes feelings of trust, safety, and emotional connection. It also reduces cortisol levels, alters hormones, and increases serotonin and dopamine levels. In other words, it is scientifically measurable that your heart (mood) state affects those around you. These findings suggest that individuals might be able to influence or resonate with others emotionally, enhancing connection and understanding.

From an evolutionary perspective, emotions developed as an immediate, powerful response to ensure survival. Fear helps us avoid danger, love bonds us to others for safety and procreation, and anger mobilizes us to defend ourselves. These emotional responses are primal and instinctual, originating in the limbic system—a part of the brain that processes emotions and predates the development of the rational neocortex. These emotions are literally woven into our DNA (deoxyribonucleic acid) and retained as cellular memories.

The limbic system processes emotional stimuli faster than the prefrontal cortex processes rational thoughts. When faced with a stimulus, the amygdala (part of the limbic system) can trigger an emotional response before the brain has had time to analyze the situation logically. This "quick reaction" mechanism ensures survival but often overrides reason. Emotional memories are stronger and longer-lasting than neutral ones because they are stored in the amygdala and hippocampus, creating deep impressions that guide future actions through memory recall.

The heart is more than a pump; it communicates with the brain and body in profound ways. The heart sends more signals to the brain than the brain sends to the heart,[14] influencing emotional experience, decision-making, and cognitive function. From a spiritual perspective, emotions may be viewed as a reflection of the soul and a conduit for divine guidance. Scripture often refers to the heart as the seat of wisdom, understanding, and connection with God. Proverbs 4:23 says, "Above all else, guard your heart, for everything you do flows from it," emphasizing the heart's primacy in directing our lives.

The Heart-Mind Connection: Exploring the Intrinsic Cardiac Nervous System's Role in Well-Being

Research over the last few decades has revealed the grander influence the heart has on physical, emotional, mental, and spiritual well-being. While the heart has long been known to have its own network of neurons, the understanding of its complexity and function has evolved significantly beyond simply innervating the heart. Investigations in the 1970s identified the presence of ganglia—clusters of nerve cell bodies that act as relay points for transmitting signals—and a complex network of neurons intertwined within cardiac tissue. Often referred to as the "heart's nervous system," this complex cardiac neural network is an active participant in the broader neuro-cardiac interactions that affect far more than just the amount of blood coursing through our blood vessels, as revealed by completed and ongoing research.

To date, research has discovered that the heart's neural network, or intrinsic cardiac nervous system, can generate its own rhythm and regulate heart function independently of the central nervous system. The heart's independence becomes more evident in conditions where the heart and brain may be compromised.[15] Recent studies indicate a compelling connection between heart function and the processing of emotional and cognitive information. Intriguingly, the heart demonstrates a form of memory that is significantly influenced by the intrinsic cardiac nervous system.[16] Researchers have found that this neural network in the heart plays a crucial role in decision-making, memory, and mood regulation.[17] Put simply, the heart has the capacity to recall past experiences and adjust its functions in response, with these memories also impacting responses from the central nervous system. Not surprisingly, this can affect HRV. For instance, repetitive stressors could lead to lasting adaptations in HRV, potentially amplifying the stress response. Research findings demonstrate neuroplasticity—the ability of neurons to change structurally and functionally in response to stimuli—within the heart, which likely involves changes in neuronal connections and neurotransmitter levels that ultimately affect the heart's response to emotional states.[18] There's even growing evidence that the function of the intrinsic cardiac nervous system may be altered in various cardiovascular diseases, which influences heart health and disease progression.[19,20] Ultimately, these insights underscore the complexity of the heart as not merely a pump but as a dynamic organ intricately connected to both emotional experiences and overall physiological well-being.

The vagus nerve is the crucial pathway for the interaction between the cardiac nervous system and the central nervous system, transmitting signals between the heart and the brain. Emotional states such as excitement, anxiety, and stress can trigger physiological responses in the heart. For example, a surge of adrenaline during a stressful situation increases heart rate and blood pressure, leading to decreased vagal tone and a greater vulnerability to stress.[21] Conversely, a relaxed state enhances vagal tone, promoting heart rate variability and overall cardiovascular health.[22] Existing and emerging research makes it abundantly clear that the intrinsic cardiac system plays a critical role not only in regulating heart function but also in processing emotional and cognitive influences.

The Quantum Connection: Energy Dynamics in DNA Interactions and Their Role in Vitality

More evidence of energy being the underpinning force of vitality is the observation that DNA strands recognize similar DNA strands from a distance and the specific paring of nitrogenous bases—adenine (A), thymine (T), cytosine (C), and guanine (G)—that make up DNA appears to be highly self-directed, almost "telepathic.".[23] So these bases pair up and bond to make new DNA in a very specific and predictable pattern, such as adenine with thymine and cytosine with guanine, not through biochemical or physical attraction as previously thought, but as directed by quantum energy. At least, that is the theory that will likely be proven in the future.

Recognition by and interactions with similar DNA strands is a process crucial for various cellular functions, including replication, repair, and regulation of gene expression. This recognition is facilitated by the structure of DNA, where complementary nitrogenous bases allow specific pairings. Some researchers speculate that energy at the quantum level facilitates this DNA recognition and interaction. In other words, energy enables non-local signaling between DNA strands without direct contact. You could envision this in the context of Bluetooth technology—a short-range wireless technology standard designed for exchanging data between devices. Through Bluetooth technology, two of your devices are able to connect and communicate without the need for cables. Your DNA uses a similar sharing of energy to pair and function efficiently. The potential that energy plays a fundamental role in DNA interactions, and therefore health and healing, is a topic of growing interest in both biological and quantum research.

To understand how DNA works, we need to think about energy and how it behaves. DNA has a special shape called a double helix, and this shape stays relatively stable because of how the parts of the DNA interact with each other and their surroundings. Things like temperature, acidity (pH), and the number of certain particles in the solution can change how these parts interact. This shows that energy is really important for keeping DNA healthy and working properly. The specific pairing of nitrogenous bases in DNA can also be viewed through the lens of energetics. The formation of hydrogen bonds (the interactions between adenine-thymine and cytosine-guanine) is energetically favorable and highly specific, effectively guiding the structure and function of the DNA molecule. This line of inquiry may provide valuable insights that bridge the gap between quantum biology, molecular genetics, and holistic health paradigms, potentially reshaping our understanding of how energy dynamics contribute to vitality and well-being.

To simplify the concept of DNA and its interactions, imagine DNA as a beautifully organized garden. The double-helix shape of DNA is like the layout of a well-designed garden, with pathways (the sugar-phosphate backbone) that help structure everything and ensure easy access to the plants. In the garden, the plants represent the nitrogenous bases (adenine, thymine, cytosine, and guanine). Each pair of plants (adenine with thymine and cytosine with guanine) has a special way of growing together, much like how the bases bond through hydrogen bonds. The stability and health of the garden depend on various environmental factors like temperature, sunlight, and moisture (pH and other particles in the solution). If the weather is just right, the plants thrive and produce beautiful flowers (healthy, functioning genes). However, if it gets too hot, too dry, or too acidic, the plants may struggle to grow properly or may even wilt. Just as the plants in the garden rely on proper sunlight, water, and nutrients to interact well and stay healthy, DNA requires optimal energy conditions (like temperature and pH) to maintain its structure and function effectively. The collaboration of these conditions allows the garden (DNA) to flourish and sustain life. By thinking of DNA as a garden, it becomes easier to visualize how its structure and function are shaped by interactions and environmental conditions. Just as a garden flourishes through the right balance of energy—sunlight, water, and soil nutrients—DNA relies on the correct energy dynamics to remain stable and perform its vital roles in life.

Harmonizing with Earth's Energies for Life and Healing

The idea that life on Earth has evolved alongside the planet's magnetic fields and Schumann resonances touches on the intricate relationship between the environment and biological systems. This concept can be beautifully woven into discussions of divine energy healing, which emphasizes the interconnectedness of life, energy, and the universe.

The Earth generates a magnetic field that extends into space and plays a crucial role in protecting the planet from solar radiation and cosmic rays. This magnetic field also creates a stable environment for many forms of life. Organisms, from migratory birds to sea turtles, have been shown to utilize Earth's magnetic field for navigation and orientation. This suggests that these natural energies are integral to their survival and behavior.

The Schumann resonances are a set of electromagnetic waves that occur in the Earth's atmosphere. These waves are created by lightning strikes and travel around the Earth between the surface and the ionosphere. The fundamental frequency of these resonances is approximately 7.83 Hz, which is thought to be in sync with the brain's alpha brainwaves. This resonance is often linked to feelings of grounding and well-being and is considered a natural rhythm that may influence our biological processes.

Divine energy as a source of life and healing emphasizes that everything in the universe is interconnected through energy. Channeling or harnessing this energy can promote healing and restoration within individuals. If life forms have evolved in harmony with Earth's natural energies, such as magnetic fields and Schumann resonances, it stands to reason that these elements can also play a role in healing practices.

Divine energy healing may involve aligning an individual's energy with the Earth's natural frequencies. There is a growing body of research suggesting that exposure to natural electromagnetic fields can have positive effects on human health and well-being.[24] For example, spending time in nature or near bodies of water can help reduce stress and improve mental clarity. Negative ions, often abundant in natural settings, like near waterfalls, forests, and beaches, are thought to have various health benefits. These ions are negatively charged molecules that arise when water molecules break apart due to the force of falling water or other natural processes. Negative ions support optimum health in many ways including regulating serotonin levels, balancing mood, reducing the effects of airborne allergens and pollutants, boosting immune activity, improving sleep quality, increasing energy and focus, and helping to neutralize free radicals. By tapping into these natural energies, individuals can restore balance and promote physical, mental, emotional, and spiritual healing.

Unlocking Our True Potential for Health, Healing, and Connection with the Divine

In conclusion, recognizing the intricate dance of energy that permeates every aspect of our being leads us to a deeper understanding of health and healing. As explored throughout this book, human health transcends mere physical well-being; it encompasses the dynamic interplay between our mental, emotional, and spiritual states, all of which are intricately connected to our energetic nature. By embracing this holistic perspective and acknowledging the profound insights provided by pioneers like Einstein and Tesla, we open the door to innovative approaches in medicine that leverage the mystique of energy as both a healing force and a source of vitality. As science advances and bridges the realms of bioenergetics, quantum biology, and modern health practices, we are reminded that true wellness emerges not just from treating symptoms, but from cultivating an awareness of how energy converges within us and the world around us. As we continue this exploration, we will uncover the life-changing potential of aligning ourselves with the natural energies of the Earth, fostering healing and harmony within ourselves and connecting to the broader tapestry of life. Each step toward understanding our energetic essence is a step toward unlocking our true potential for health, healing, and connection with the Divine.

Nikola Tesla's Radiant Energy Concept

Nikola Tesla believed a form of energy could be harnessed from the environment, particularly from the sun, cosmic rays, and atmospheric electricity. The concept of radiant energy, as described by Nikola Tesla, and divine or healing energy share some interesting parallels.

Tesla's theory of energy that exists all around us parallels the concept of a divine energy—an all-pervasive energy that flows through everything. Tesla's belief that energy is omnipresent, dynamic, and potentially healing if harnessed correctly aligns with divine energy. He even suggested that his work was inspired by deeper universal truths, sometimes hinting at higher intelligence or divine design behind energy itself.

Tesla himself did not directly link his radiant energy to the source of healing, but he did explore electromagnetic healing technologies:

- Tesla Coils & Electrotherapy. Tesla experimented with high-frequency currents for potential healing benefits.
- Pulsed Electromagnetic Fields (PEMFs). A modern extension of Tesla's work, used for cellular healing, pain relief, and bone regeneration.
- Violet Ray Devices. Early healing devices inspired by Tesla's electrical work, used for improving circulation and reducing inflammation.

While mainstream science sees Tesla's radiant energy as a physical phenomenon, many believe it could also interact with human bioenergetic fields. If energy is fundamental to all existence, then physical, mental, and spiritual well-being could be influenced by how we harness and balance it.

CHAPTER TWO

Divine Energy, Stress, Emotions, and Cellular Memory

In an era where the frenzied pace of life often overwhelms our senses, it becomes increasingly crucial to explore the deep connection between our emotional states, physiological responses, and the intricate workings of our cellular memory. Research illuminates the profound impact that achieving emotional and physiological coherence can have on our overall well-being. Imagine the harmony of a finely tuned orchestra, where each instrument plays its part with precision, guiding the melody toward a beautiful symphony. Just as a skilled conductor ensures every musician syncs seamlessly, our bodies rely on the collective cooperation of cells, tissues, and organs to maintain balance and optimal health. This chapter delves into how stress and emotions influence not only our immediate health but also leave lasting imprints within our cellular architecture, shaping our responses to life for generations to come. By understanding this interplay, we can harness the power of divine energy to cultivate resilience and foster healing, ultimately transforming our lives into a harmonious melody of vitality and connection.

Understanding Emotional and Physiological Coherence Through Heart Rate Variability

Research from institutions like the HeartMath Institute suggests that achieving emotional and physiological coherence (harmonized energy between the heart and brain, or put another way, the heart, mind, and emotions) can promote healing and well-being. To visualize biological coherence, we can draw parallels to a finely tuned orchestra. Within a well-trained professional orchestra, each instrument harmoniously contributes to the greater musical composition. Every musician, no matter how skilled, must play their part with precision, awareness, and synchronization, adhering to the conductor's guidance. If even one instrument plays out of tune or loses the rhythm, it disrupts the entire ensemble, creating discord. In the same way, biological coherence relies on the harmonious interplay between various systems in the body—cells, tissues, organs, and the signals they exchange, under the direction of the Master Conductor. A finely tuned orchestra and the coherent body share the same principles: balance, harmony, and purposeful interaction. By striving for coherence, we can ensure that our "orchestra" plays the most beautiful and harmonious symphony of life.

One of the key tests that the HeartMath Institute relies upon for evaluating physiological coherence is heart rate variability (HRV). This is largely because they believe that the heart is more than a pump for blood but also plays a critical role in emotional experience and decision-making, positing that we can harness our heart's guidance to improve emotional health. They are correct in this belief, since the heart communicates with the brain through neural pathways, hormones, and even electromagnetic fields, influencing emotional experiences and cognitive processes. Individuals with impaired emotional processing—such as those with damage to areas of the brain involved in emotional evaluation—often struggle with making decisions. This indicates that emotions, influenced by physiological state and the heart's cues, are integral to the decision-making process. Emotional responses (heart) often guide our choices, even omitting reason (brain) because emotions are tied to survival, especially under situations of uncertainty or rapid judgment.

HRV is a key indicator of nervous system coherence because it reflects the dynamic interplay between the sympathetic (fight-or-flight) and parasympathetic (rest-and-digest) branches of the autonomic nervous system. HRV measures the variation in time between heartbeats. Imagine your heart is a drummer in a band. Sometimes it beats fast, like during a drum solo, and sometimes it beats slow, like during a quiet song. The way your heart changes its beat is called HRV. Higher HRV is linked to greater emotional regulation and awareness. Understanding this intricate interplay between the heart and brain can lead to better emotional awareness and more informed decision-making processes.

The heart's rhythm is intricately balanced by various factors, such as the autonomic nervous system, breathing patterns, hormonal influences, and other physiological processes. This dynamic interplay suggests that the heart, guided by divine energy, should adapt and display enhanced complexity over different time intervals, reflecting its responsiveness to these interconnected systems. When the body is under stress, the sympathetic nervous system dominates, leading to less variability in heart rate as the body prepares for action. In contrast, during relaxed states, the parasympathetic nervous system prevails, allowing for increased variability in heart rate.

Scientists can measure HRV in different ways. One way is by looking at the frequency of the heartbeats, kind of like counting the beats per minute. They look at how often the heart speeds up and slows down. By measuring these frequencies, scientists can learn a lot about your overall health. Another way to analyze HRV is by looking at what happens in different "frequency bands," which are basically groups of heart rate changes that happen at certain speeds. Here are the key parts:

- *Power spectrum analysis.* Scientists use special math to break down heart rate data into different speeds or "frequencies." This tells us how much change happens at those different speeds.
- *Frequency bands.*
  - ☐ Low Frequency (LF) reflects how both our sympathetic nervous system (which speeds us up) and parasympathetic nervous system (which calms us down) are working. LF is like the steady drumbeat in the background. It is a measure of how well your body is managing stress.
  - ☐ High Frequency (HF) mainly shows how our body's calming system (the parasympathetic system) is working, especially when we breathe. HF is like the quick drum rolls. It shows how quickly your heart can respond to changes, like when you stand up or exercise.
  - ☐ Very Low Frequency (VLF) and Ultra-Low Frequency (ULF) bands are less understood but might relate to long-term body functions like breathing and sleeping.
- *LF/HF ratio.* This is a simple number that compares the LF and HF bands. If the number is high, it means we might be more stressed; if it's low, it means we might be calmer.
- *Total power.* This is a measure of all the heart rate changes together, showing the overall activity of our heart.
- *Normalized units.* Scientists also use normalized units (like LFnu and HFnu) to see how much of the heart

activity comes from the sympathetic versus the parasympathetic systems.

Measuring HRV can help doctors see how well our body is managing stress and working overall. It also helps us understand our emotions and how our body reacts to them. Additionally, athletes use it to understand if they need to rest or train harder based on how their body is responding. In short, HRV gives us important clues about our health and how our body responds to everyday life. In the context of divine energy, it is a physiological measure of how coherent divine energy is in your body and your body's current healing potential.

Higher HRV is associated with superior physiological resilience and health, while lower HRV is a sign of current or future health problems because it indicates poor physiological resilience. Studies conducted by the HeartMath Institute suggest that achieving physiological coherence through various methods (e.g., breathing exercises) reduces stress and anxiety, thus improving overall health..[25] Essentially, disconnecting from the perpetual "fight-or-flight" response that modern humans are trapped in allows the body to perform its function as the true healer and restore vigor and homeostasis.

The Chronic Stress Epidemic: Unpacking the Hypothalamic-Pituitary-Adrenal Axis and Its Impact on Health

Substantial research indicates that many people in modern society experience a chronic state of mild to moderate psychological stress. Fast-paced lifestyles, economic uncertainty, technological overload, social pressures, and a smorgasbord of environmental stressors create the perfect storm for our stress response to be continuously active. This is less than ideal considering the demonstrable adverse effects of chronic stress in humans, including macroscopic changes in brain structure, increased inflammation, neuroendocrine and immune imbalances, cardiovascular disease, and depression.[26] In fact, some sources suggest that ninety percent or more of all diseases are stress-related.[27,28] One cannot naively dismiss stress as a causative factor in much of ill health, nor ignore stress and achieve optimum wellness.

To understand this connection between stress, emotions, and health, we need to explore the stress response and the role of the hypothalamic-pituitary-adrenal axis (HPAA). The stress response is a complex physiological and psychological mechanism that prepares the body to handle perceived threats or challenges. At the center of this response is the HPAA, a critical system that regulates stress hormones and orchestrates the body's response to stressors.

When you perceive a threat—whether physical, emotional, or environmental—your body activates its stress response. This process is referred to as the "fight-or-flight" response and is characterized by a series of physiological changes that prepare the body to either confront or flee from the perceived danger. These changes include increased heart rate, heightened blood pressure, rapid breathing, and dilation of the pupils. Additionally, the body diverts blood away from non-essential functions, such as digestion, and increases blood flow to the muscles and brain, enabling faster physical response and heightened alertness.

The HPAA consists of three main components: the hypothalamus, the pituitary gland, and the adrenal glands. Each component plays a pivotal role in the stress response.

Located at the base of the brain, the hypothalamus acts as the command center for the body's stress response. In response to a stressor, the hypothalamus releases corticotropin-releasing hormone (CRH) into the bloodstream. This hormone signals the pituitary gland to initiate the next phase of the stress response.

The pituitary gland, often considered the "master gland" due to its regulatory influence on other endocrine glands, responds to CRH by releasing adrenocorticotropic hormone (ACTH). ACTH enters circulation, traveling to the adrenal glands.

The adrenal glands, situated on top of the kidneys, are responsible for producing and releasing various hormones, including cortisol, adrenaline (epinephrine), and norepinephrine. In the stress response, ACTH stimulates the adrenal glands to produce cortisol, a primary stress hormone.

Cortisol plays a crucial role in the body's response to stress. It helps mobilize energy by increasing glucose levels in the bloodstream through gluconeogenesis (the production of glucose from non-carbohydrate sources) and by breaking down fat and protein stores. This provides the body with the energy needed for an immediate response. During chronic stress, the body's continuous reliance on this energy mobilization mechanism can lead to several negative consequences, including metabolic imbalance—such as insulin resistance and metabolic syndrome, persistent inflammation, suppressed immune function, anxiety, depression, cognitive impairment, muscle tension, cardiovascular disease, and gastrointestinal issues. While acute cortisol release can enhance the immune response in the short term, prolonged exposure to elevated cortisol levels can suppress immune function, increasing vulnerability to infections. Cortisol promotes sodium retention and potassium excretion, helping maintain blood pressure and fluid balance during stressful situations. However, chronic, elevated cortisol levels can lead to electrolyte imbalances in the long term. Cortisol influences cognitive functions, such as memory, attention, and decision-making. During acute stress, cognitive processes may enhance focus and awareness, but chronic stress and prolonged cortisol exposure can impair cognitive performance and contribute to anxiety and depression. If you are stressed all the time, even mild, practically imperceivable stress, your body keeps pumping out cortisol. When this happens, you can experience sleep disturbances, stomach pain, get sick more often, or experience a whole host of undesirable symptoms.

The HPAA also operates under a feedback loop—a biological mechanism that regulates a system by responding to changes within that system—to prevent overactivation. Elevated cortisol levels signal the hypothalamus and pituitary gland to decrease the production of CRH and ACTH, effectively reducing cortisol secretion from the adrenal glands. This negative feedback loop is essential for maintaining homeostasis and ensuring that the body does not remain in a heightened state of alertness indefinitely. While the stress response is an adaptive mechanism that can protect individuals in the short term, chronic activation of the HPAA due to prolonged stress can have deleterious effects on the body and mind.

Sustained stress may result in a hyperactive HPAA, characterized by consistently elevated levels of cortisol. This state can contribute to various health issues, including obesity, hypertension, diabetes, cardiovascular disease, and mental health disorders such as anxiety and depression. Over time, the body may become desensitized to cortisol, leading to an impaired ability to respond to new stressors. This can hinder the body's recovery mechanisms and exacerbate stress-related health challenges. Chronic stress is also associated with structural and functional changes in the brain, particularly in areas such as the hippocampus, amygdala, and prefrontal cortex. These changes can impact mood regulation, memory, and decision-making processes.

Understanding the intricacies of the HPAA and its role in the stress response is crucial for developing effective interventions and promoting health and well-being in the face of stress. There's a growing body of evidence linking trauma to chronic health issues. For instance, individuals who have experienced traumatic events are more susceptible to conditions such as autoimmune diseases, heart disease, and obesity.[29,30,31] Some researchers argue that these physical conditions may stem from the unresolved emotional pain held in the body—suggesting that the mind and body are interconnected in astonishing ways.

Epigenetic Footprints: How Stress and Trauma Shape Gene Expression Across Generations

As mentioned earlier, when we experience stress, our bodies release hormones such as cortisol. These hormones can affect how our genes work. They can turn certain genes on or off or up or down, which can change how our cells function. This is called epigenetic modification, which is the alteration of the expression of genes without producing changes to the DNA sequence. Think of this like a dimmer switch for your genes. Stress can turn up or down the activity of certain genes, affecting how they work. Over time, these changes can build up and affect our health. This means that life experiences can alter how our genes are turned on or off, potentially influencing our health for generations.

Our cells remember the stress we've experienced, and this memory can influence our future health and the future health of our offspring. Emerging research suggests that traumatic experiences experienced by your ancestors can indeed be passed down through generations. This phenomenon is often linked to epigenetics. For example, researchers found that Holocaust exposure influenced FKBP5 methylation—a stress gene linked to post-traumatic stress disorder (PTSD), depression, and mood and anxiety disorders.[32] This was observed in parents exposed to the horrors of concentration camps, as well as their offspring. Essentially, children born to parents who survived the Holocaust had different stress hormone profiles caused by epigenetic changes that made them more prone to anxiety disorders.

Other evidence linking the passage of altered gene expression to subsequent generations without these generations being directly exposed to the trauma can be found in the offspring of individuals who experienced racial trauma. Evidence strongly indicates that environmental-induced epigenetic changes can lead to lasting transgenerational effects.[33] Specifically, the research shows that offspring of those who experienced racial trauma share different anxiety and adaptive survival behaviors. Cellular retention and epigenetics may be responsible for a legacy of trauma sometimes seen in families.

Cellular Memory: The Legacy of Trauma and Emotion in Shaping Health

These findings touch on a fascinating idea: cellular memory. Not only can our cells retain memories of past experiences, traumas, and even feelings, but these cellular memories can be passed down through generations and potentially impact the physical and emotional health of these future generations.

At its core, the idea suggests that our cells are not just passively responding to physiological needs and signals; rather, they are active participants in our life story. Every experience we go through—whether it is joyful or traumatic—may leave traces in our cells, influencing how we feel and how our body functions. In 1992, Sara Paddison (now Sara Childre), the president of the HeartMath Institute, proposed that maintaining an underlying state of unconditional love promotes a coherent biofield that is responsible for maintaining homeostasis and promoting health in general..[34] This is an interesting thought that suggests that only people who can generate a genuine state of unconditional love may be able to resonate with cells and DNA itself to modulate their state. Further supporting this hypothesis, cell biologist Dr. Glen Rein even showed that having people hold test tubes containing DNA while attempting to create a healing environment triggered conformational changes in the DNA.[35] This perspective not only elevates our understanding of the intricate connections between emotions, cellular biology, and overall health but also invites us to explore the profound impact of love and positive intentions on our very biology. By recognizing our role as co-creators of our health and well-being, we empower ourselves to cultivate environments—both internal and external—that foster healing and harmony, ultimately leading to a more profound and holistic approach to wellness.

To better understand conformation changes in DNA, imagine DNA as a twisted ladder. While it usually maintains this classic double-helix shape, it can sometimes change its form. These changes, known as conformational changes, are crucial for various cellular processes.

Common DNA conformations:

- B-DNA. This is the most common form, the classic double-helix.
- A-DNA. A slightly more compact form, often found in dehydrated DNA or DNA-RNA hybrids.
- Z-DNA. A left-handed helix, different from the right-handed B-DNA. It can form in certain DNA sequences, particularly those with alternating purines and pyrimidines.

Changes in DNA conformation matter for a variety of reasons:

- Gene regulation. Proteins can bind to DNA in specific conformations, activating or repressing gene expression.
- DNA replication and repair. Enzymes involved in these processes need to interact with DNA, and sometimes conformational changes are necessary.
- Chromatin structure. The way DNA is packaged within chromosomes involves various levels of coiling and folding, influenced by DNA conformation.

In essence, DNA's ability to change shape is a fundamental aspect of its function. These conformational changes allow for a wide range of biological processes and are essential for life.

So, it may not be the genetics you inherited from your parents, but the cellular memories or epigenetics that they passed on that are driving certain health outcomes. This is why it is important to manage stress, recognize and deal with generational distress and adversity, and find healthy ways to overcome them. Understanding cellular memory can empower us to take a comprehensive approach to health. Instead of simply treating physical symptoms, we can acknowledge and address the emotional and psychological roots of our conditions.

It is important to understand that cellular memory does not imply that any health issue is solely the result of personal trauma or emotional experiences. Lifestyle, environment, toxic burden, and to a lesser extent genetics, also play significant roles. As we continue to explore the intersection of psychology, biology, and health, one thing becomes clear: taking a holistic approach to our well-being can be a transformative step toward achieving a healthier, more balanced life.

Unlocking the Path to Emotional and Physical Healing Through Coherence

The interaction between psychological processes, the nervous system, and the immune system suggests a strong connection between the mind's energy and physical health. Emotional states carry a form of "energy" in the form of neural and biochemical signals that impact physical health.[36,37] When your emotional and physiological states are synchronized, the body operates more efficiently and performs its healing responsibilities at a higher level.

In understanding the profound connection between mind, emotions, body, and spirit, it becomes evident that achieving emotional and physiological coherence is not merely a concept but a tangible pathway to healing and wholeness. The interplay between our stress responses, cellular memories, and genetic expression reveals how deeply interconnected our life experiences are with our physical health. By recognizing the role of the heart in guiding emotional resilience and embracing practices that promote coherence—like mindfulness, prayer, or breathwork—we empower our bodies to function as the remarkable healers they are designed to be. This comprehensive approach allows us to address not only the symptoms of imbalance but also the underlying emotional and spiritual roots, fostering a life of harmony, vitality, and lasting well-being. In this light, healing transcends the physical, becoming a sacred journey of transformation that unites us with our true selves and the divine energy that sustains us.

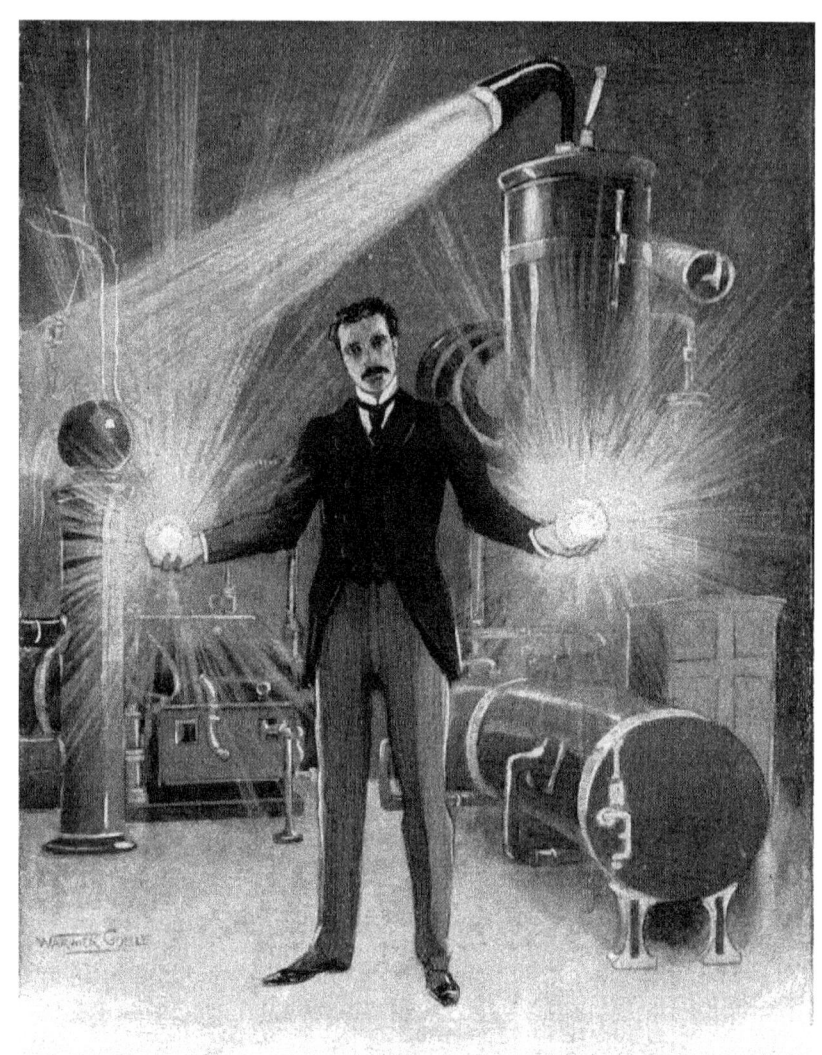

Nikola Tesla holding in his hands balls of flame

CHAPTER THREE

The Body is the Divinely Designed Healer

One thing that needs to be made absolutely clear is that the body is always the healer, not anything you do, apply, or take. While good nutrition, exercise, stress management, proper sleep, reducing toxic load, healthy relationships, smart supplementation, and essential oils each play a role in your health, in the end, these only support or hinder the innate healing abilities of the body. What does the body use to maintain and restore health? Divine energy!

The Miraculous Self-Healing Body

The body is divinely designed with multiple complex systems, mechanisms, and pathways that work synergistically to maintain health, adapt to challenges, and promote healing. It does so marvelously most of the time. But as we neglect our lifestyle or are exposed to toxins, its healing potential diminishes and health declines.

Proof of our self-healing mechanisms can be found in our remarkable ability to regenerate tissues and organs. Cells within the skin renew every 28 to 40 days, the liver can regenerate damaged tissue within a few weeks, and the intestinal lining renews every few days. This inherent resilience not only highlights the body's capability to restore itself but also underscores the complex biological processes that support healing. Furthermore, understanding these regenerative capabilities encourages us to engage in practices that promote overall health, such as proper nutrition and stress management. Ultimately, embracing our natural healing potential can empower us to live healthier, more vibrant lives.

Skin cells renew in a layered process that involves cell division, migration, maturation, and shedding. New cells are created at the deepest layer (basal layer). These cells gradually move upwards through the layers of the skin. As they rise, they flatten and fill with a tough protein called keratin. Once they reach the surface, they become dead skin cells and are shed. This constant cycle ensures a fresh protective outer layer.

Your skin is a protective suit and barrier. It has a remarkable ability to maintain this barrier. When you get a cut, it is like a tiny hole in your suit. Your body is intelligent and knows how to heal the cut. First, it sends special cells to the cut to clean it up. Then, it sends other cells to patch up the hole. These cells work hard to weave together new skin, just like sewing a rip in your clothes. As the new skin grows, it gets stronger and stronger until the cut is completely healed and your skin is affords full protected again.

Liver regeneration is a remarkable process where the liver can repair itself after damage. When part of the liver is removed or injured, the remaining liver cells proliferate, differentiate, and regrow. During proliferation, liver cells begin to multiply rapidly. These new cells mature into different liver cell types (differentiation). Finally, the liver tissue grows back to its original size and function. This process is regulated by a complex network of growth factors and signaling pathways.

The gastrointestinal lining is constantly renewing itself. Stem cells located in the crypts of the intestinal lining divide rapidly, producing new cells that migrate upwards, maturing as they go.

Once they reach the surface, they are shed, making way for a fresh layer. This rapid turnover protects the delicate gut lining from damage and ensures efficient nutrient absorption.

Other signs of our self-healing body include immune surveillance and the continual management of toxic burden. Immune surveillance remains vigilant to detect and neutralize pathogens and abnormal cells to prevent disease. This is like having a security system that constantly patrols your body, looking for anything suspicious. Immune cells are the guards of this system, and when they find something harmful, they attack and destroy it, protecting you from infection and disease. Organs like the liver, kidneys, colon, lungs, and lymphatic system process and eliminate toxins efficiently under normal conditions. Your liver, the major organ of detoxification, acts like a filter processing and breaking down toxins into less harmful substances. Then, your kidneys filter your blood, removing the waste products and excess water. These waste products, along with the processed toxins from your liver, are turned into urine. Your lungs help with the cleansing process by removing carbon dioxide and other harmful substances you breathe in. Your intestines help eliminate solid waste containing undigested food and other waste products, including some toxins, from your body. Finally, the lymphatic system collects excess fluid from tissues containing cellular waste products that are removed from the body. These adaptive systems ensure survival and continued healthy function.

The Weighty Impact of Lifestyle and Environment on Self-Healing

However, poor lifestyle choices profoundly influence the intrinsic ability of the body to maintain health. A nutrient-deficient diet impairs energy production—remember all cells require energy to function—hampers immune surveillance, and interferes with cellular repair. Overconsumption of processed foods, a common occurrence in Westernized cultures, leads to chronic inflammation and metabolic dysfunction. Sedentary behavior disrupts cardiovascular health, impairs lymphatic flow, and weakens or misaligns musculoskeletal integrity. Persistent stress exhausts the HPAA, reduces immune competence, and accelerates aging. Sleep deprivation hinders cellular repair, brain detoxification (via the glymphatic system), and hormone balance. While the body's healing ability is extraordinary and infinite, it thrives best in an environment supported by a healthy lifestyle. Your divine energy requires a healthy landscape to perform efficiently.

Modern environments expose you to a range of toxins that burden the body. Heavy metals (e.g., mercury, lead) and chemicals (e.g., pesticides, herbicides, phthalates) accumulate in tissues, disrupting cellular function and hormone signaling. Antibiotics, poor diet, inactivity, and chemicals disrupt the gut microbiome, which plays a crucial role in digestion, immunity, and mental health. Toxins increase the production of free radicals, resulting in cellular damage and reduced healing capacity. While not well accepted by Western medicine, the available evidence suggests that your toxic load plays a huge role in your overall health. The path to restoration and healing begins by establishing a terrain (healthy body) where healing divine energy is ubiquitous, permitting the body's remarkable capacity for recovery to shine.

Divine Design: Embracing the Awe and Complexity of Creation in the Human Body

The intricate interplay of body systems points to a divine design that is both awe-inspiring and humbling. It is highly problematic to dismiss a higher intelligence in our creation when you consider the body's ability to self-regulate and heal. Every cell, tissue, and organ, working in harmonious symphony, reveals a complexity that defies chance. From the delicate dance of neurons in the brain to the rhythmic beat of the heart, each component plays a vital role in sustaining life.

Consider the homeostasis maintained by our endocrine system, which intricately regulates hormones to balance metabolism, growth, and stress response. The feedback loops between glands such as the pituitary, thyroid, and adrenal glands demonstrate a finely tuned communication network essential for survival. Even more remarkable is the immune system, a sophisticated defense mechanism designed to recognize and neutralize pathogens and other threats, showcasing both adaptability and specificity that ensures our protection.

Furthermore, the digestive system exemplifies this divine orchestration, with its multitude of processes—from the mechanical breakdown of food in the stomach to the absorption of vital nutrients in the intestines—each stage is essential to our overall well-being. The microbiome, a community of trillions of microbes that cohabitate with us, collaborates intimately with our digestive and immune systems, further highlighting an elaborate interplay crucial to health and nutrition.

Consider the miracle of sight as an example of divine creation. The intricate structure of the eye, with its lens, cornea, and retina, captures and processes light, allowing us to perceive the beauty of the world around us. The brain, a marvel of neural networks, interprets these visual signals, enabling us to recognize faces, read, and appreciate art. The human eye is far more complex than the most advanced cameras made by man. Human sight arises from a combination of sophisticated anatomical structures, intricate biochemical processes, advanced neural circuitry, and high-level cognitive functions. The possibility that the eye formed by chance or evolution without divine involvement is extremely remote.

Nevertheless, the idea of divine creation must first be grounded in faith, and then, as we exercise faith in this eternal truth, our conviction in divine creation grows increasingly stronger. Recognizing the breathtaking intricacies of the human body not only compels us to appreciate the wonders of our existence but also invites us to engage with these systems mindfully, nurturing them with respect and reverence.

God's Divine Energy as the Ultimate Healer

The human body is a marvel of engineering, designed for both strength and resilience. The intricate design of the human body is a masterpiece that inspires awe and wonder, inviting us to contemplate the divine intelligence that brought it into existence. Its current terrestrial state is not designed to live on forever, but in a future time, a change will occur in the human body for it to thrive indefinitely.

The body of research demonstrates that the mind and body are inextricably linked, and energy—whether biochemical, electromagnetic, or emotional—plays a significant role in regulating health. This divine energy exercised by the body is therefore the ultimate source of human healing, and discovering ways to harness it will lead to an evolution in human healing beyond our wildest ambitions.

CHAPTER FOUR

What is Divine Energy?

During His mortal ministry, Jesus Christ healed the sick, caused the lame to walk, gave sight to the blind, opened the ears of the deaf, and even raised the dead. His disciples performed similar miracles using the same power and authority which He bestowed on them. The power or force by which Christ healed and raised the dead, and subsequently entrusted to His disciples, is not fully understood nor measurable by current science, but it is a real force. In fact, it is the divine energy or power that comes from God through Christ that gives life and light to all things—also known as the Light of Christ. It is the light found in all things and by which all things are governed. Without it, there would be no life.

Light: Fundamentally Woven into the Fabric of Life

Light is fundamentally woven into the fabric of life, serving as a critical energy source that sustains and nurtures all living things. This vital force influences a myriad of biological processes, highlighting its importance across different life forms.

For plants, light is essential for photosynthesis, the process through which they convert sunlight into chemical energy. Chlorophyll in plant cells absorbs light energy, primarily from the blue and red parts of the spectrum and uses it to transform carbon dioxide and water into glucose and oxygen. This process not only fuels the plant's growth and development but also produces the oxygen necessary for the survival of aerobic organisms, including humans. Thus, light serves as the bedrock of food webs, supporting life on Earth.

In humans, light plays a pivotal role in regulating circadian rhythms, the intrinsic biological clock that governs the sleep-wake cycle and various physiological processes throughout the day. Exposure to natural light, particularly in the morning, helps synchronize our internal clocks, promoting alertness and well-being. Conversely, artificial light, especially blue light emitted by screens, can disrupt these rhythms, leading to sleep disturbances and various health issues. This interplay between light and our biological systems underlines how vital it is for our mental and physical health.

Light also impacts mood and perception, with sunlight being linked to the production of serotonin, a neurotransmitter that contributes to feelings of happiness and well-being. Seasonal changes in daylight can influence mood disorders—such as Seasonal Affective Disorder (SAD)—which further demonstrates how closely intertwined our emotional states are with light exposure.

In the broader biosphere, light shapes ecosystems and influences animal behaviors as well. Many animals navigate their environment using light cues, and species such as migratory birds rely on celestial navigation. The presence or absence of light informs mating behaviors, feeding patterns, and even territorial claims in various species.

In essence, light is not just a source of energy; it is a vital force that promotes growth, regulates biological rhythms, and connects all living organisms in an intricate web of life. Without light, the delicate balance sustaining ecosystems would unravel, underscoring its role as an essential element of life that nurtures, sustains, and enriches the interconnected tapestry of existence.

The Spiritual Gifts of Faith and Healing

Both the faith to be healed and the faith to heal are gifts of the Spirit, exercised by both men and women through faith..[38] Spiritual gifts are received by faithful individuals from God through the Holy Ghost. Healing occurs by virtue of faith in Christ.

The concept of healing in this context is not limited to physical restoration but encompasses emotional, mental, and spiritual healing as well. The faith to be healed acknowledges the power of divine intervention in one's life. It requires an openness to believe that healing is possible, as well as trust in a higher purpose. This faith can manifest in various forms, such as prayer, worship, or acts of devotion, and it reflects a deep relationship with God—one that fosters hope and resilience even in the face of adversity.

The faith to heal, on the other hand, is a call to action. It emphasizes the importance of believers stepping into their roles as instruments of healing. This could take many forms, from offering prayers for others to providing practical support or guidance in times of need. The healing power associated with this faith underscores the biblical principle that believers are called to serve one another, reflecting Christ's compassion and love. The act of healing is not just a physical transformation; it can bring about emotional liberation, foster reconciliation, and restore broken relationships. In reality, the healing power of Christ heals all things!

Healing occurs by virtue of faith in Christ. This indicates a relational aspect in which faith is directed toward Jesus as the source of all healing. It is through His sacrifice and resurrection that we find hope for restoration. Christ's teachings and actions during His earthly ministry serve as a model for how healing unfolds—rooted in compassion, love, and the establishment of faith-filled relationships.

Moreover, this partnership with the Holy Spirit underscores the need for divine assistance in both receiving and administering healing. The Spirit empowers individuals, guiding them in their faith journeys, and providing the necessary wisdom and insight to discern how best to minister to others. This gift is not limited to a select few, as both men and women are called to partake in this divine flow of healing.

Understanding these gifts encourages a communal approach to faith, where followers of Christ support one another, pray for one another, and collectively seek healing in various forms. It fosters a spirit of unity and collaboration, urging the community to live out Christ's command to love one another.

Ultimately, the interplay of faith in healing—whether through seeking it for oneself or bestowing it upon another—demonstrates a beautiful cycle of grace and empowerment. Each act of faith, both in asking for healing and in extending healing to others, reflects the boundless love of God and the transformative power of the Holy Spirit. In this way, healing becomes not only a personal experience but a communal journey toward wholeness and restoration in Christ.

The Healing Potential of Prayer and Faith

Evidence of accessing divine energy for healing can be found in research evaluating prayer and faith healing. Millions of people worldwide believe in the power of prayer, both personal and intercessory (petitioning God for the needs and concerns of others), to heal, and even lead to miracles. A systemic review published in 2007 concluded that there was a "small, but significant, effect size for the use of intercessory prayer."[39] In other words, evaluation of the seventeen studies included in the review, most of which were randomized blinded studies, suggested that prayer can have a healing effect. More specifically, people who received intercessory prayer experienced significant improvements in their health compared to those who received standard treatment only in seven of the seventeen studies. Additionally, five more of the studies showed a trend favoring the prayer group, indicating that over seventy percent of the studies demonstrated possible or significant positive impact of prayer on healing.

A Cochrane Database systemic review from the same year that reviewed ten studies and included 7,646 people concluded it was difficult to determine the effects of prayer conclusively but that "the evidence presented so far is interesting enough to justify further study into the human aspects of the effects of prayer."[40] While the scientific evidence for the health benefits of prayer is inconclusive, this is true of nearly all things involving spirituality. God expects His children to exercise faith before receiving a witness that what they have placed their faith in is true.

All things, even the Earth we live on, were created spiritually before they were created physically.[41] There were spirit men, spirit animals, spirit plants, all things existed as spirits or spirit beings before they were physically placed upon the Earth.[42] Some interpretations of quantum physics suggest that all matter, including human beings, is composed of energy at a fundamental level. This idea can be abstractly correlated with spiritual beliefs that hypothesize humans are reflections of divine energy.

Energy Healing and Compatibility with Christianity

Instinctively touching an injured part of our body is a common human behavior that can be understood through various psychological and physiological lenses. Touching an injured area can provide a soothing effect. The act of gentle pressure or touch can stimulate sensory nerves, potentially distracting the brain from pain signals. This is related to the "gate control theory" of pain, which proposes that non-painful input (like touch) can close the gates to painful input, thus mitigating the perception of pain.

Touching a painful area can serve as a form of self-soothing, similar to how we might hug ourselves or rock back and forth when feeling distressed. This instinctive behavior can reduce stress and anxiety associated with pain. By touching the injured area, we enhance our awareness of the body's condition and foster a connection to that part of ourselves. This mindful attention can promote healing as it encourages a caring attitude toward our own body.

Perhaps another reason we intuitively and unconsciously lay hands on areas of our body that require healing is that the "laying on of hands" reinforces the belief that touch can facilitate recovery, both emotionally and physically. This loving touch can help facilitate the flow of energy within the body, promoting healing and restoration. It highlights our innate ability to connect with ourselves in times of distress and may play a role in the broader process of recovery and healing, demonstrating the profound relationship between mind, body, and spirit.

Energy healing, particularly in the context of practices like laying on of hands, shares thematic and scriptural overlaps with Christian teachings. In the New Testament, laying on of hands is a method through which healing and blessings are imparted. This ritual signifies the transfer of spiritual energy or life force. Mark 16:18 states, "they shall lay hands on the sick, and they shall recover." Similarly, Paul used this healing procedure as revealed in Acts 28:8: "And it came to pass, that the father of Publius lay sick of a fever and a bloody flux: to whom Paul entered in, and prayed, and laid his hands on him, and healed him."

Christianity teaches that God is the source of all healing and power, aligning with the idea that healing energies can be channeled through a practitioner. James 5:14-15 confirms this with these words, "Is any sick among you? let him call for the elders of the church; and let them pray over him, anointing him with oil in the name of the Lord: And the prayer of faith shall save the sick, and the Lord shall raise him up." This verse emphasizes how faith and prayer are instrumental in the healing process.

Energy healing practices often require the recipient's belief in healing, drawing parallel to the Christian belief that faith is integral to receiving God's gifts of healing. In Matthew 9:22, we read about a woman who had suffered from a disease of the blood for twelve years—that medicine of the time was unable to cure—receiving healing simply though faith and by touching the hem of Christ's garment. It states, "But Jesus turned him about, and when he saw her, he said, 'Daughter, be of good comfort; thy faith hath made thee whole.' And the woman was made whole from that hour." This emphasizes that faith can be a conduit for healing, similar to how energy healing methodologies often require a focused intention from the recipient.

The New Testament speaks about spiritual gifts, including healing, which aligns with the notion of energy healing as a divine gift that can be shared and utilized for others' benefit. In the famous treatise on gifts of the Spirit attributed to Paul, 1 Corinthians 12:9 states, "To another faith by the same Spirit; to another gift of healing by the same Spirit." This verse suggests that healing is a spiritual gift, showing harmony with the idea that practitioners can channel energy for healing purposes.

While traditional Christianity may not explicitly endorse energy healing as it is understood in modern practices, the principles of laying on of hands and the emphasis on divine healing and spiritual gifts create a framework where energy healing concepts can find compatibility. The biblical references provide a foundation for exploring how the transfer of spiritual energy—whether through prayer, laying on of hands, or other means—can be viewed as congruent with Christian beliefs about healing and divine intervention.

The Flow of Divine Energy: Understanding Healing Through Biophotons

Although not fully understood or measurable, it can be theorized that the power by which all things were created is divine energy. And this divine energy is also harnessed by the body to promote all healing. Each living thing created by God has this divine energy flowing in, through, and around it. Divine energy (the Light of Christ) is in the sun, the moon, the stars, everything in the universe, and the power by which all these things were created. It is the law by which all things in Heaven and Earth are governed.[43] It is the source of life as we know it. Knowing that divine energy created all things helps us understand how it can be harnessed to heal what it has created.

Biophotons are tiny particles of light that are emitted by living organisms, including humans. They were first discovered in the 1920s by German physicist Fritz Popp, who demonstrated that living cells emit light in response to various stimuli, such as stress, injury, or even thought patterns. Biophotons are thought to play a crucial role in maintaining cellular health, influencing gene expression, and even facilitating communication between cells.

Is it possible that biophotons are manifestations of this divine energy or a cellular response to divine energy? Or are we witnessing a dynamic exchange between divine energy and biophotons? Biophotons may even correspond to metaphysical and spiritual concepts of energy flow in the body and carry a specific vibrational frequency that corresponds to the health and vitality of biological systems. At the very least, biophotons represent a complex interaction between oxidative processes, low-energy light, and divine energy. Lifestyle behaviors—good nutrition, mindful movement, meditation—can nourish the body and raise the vibration of the individual, corresponding to balanced divine energy.

The natural world is governed by laws of physics, biology, and chemistry—both known and unknown, which maintain balance in ecosystems, planetary movements, and the universe itself. Natural cycles—day and night, the changing seasons, life and death—illustrate a divine rhythm that sustains balance in creation. Each phase has its purpose, contributing to the greater harmony of life. The coexistence of light and dark, joy and sorrow, activity and rest, male and female, and other dualities reflects the idea of divine balance. Such dualities contribute to completeness and teach dependence on God for maintaining harmony. The Earth and its systems have remarkable capacities for self-regulation and healing, such as forests regrowing after fires or rivers cleansing themselves. These processes reflect a divine mechanism of restoration.

The same is true for the human body and all of its intricate and complex workings. Human bodies are designed to heal wounds, fight infections, and recover from stress, showcasing God's balance in creation. The ability of organisms to maintain internal stability—such as temperature, pH levels, and metabolic processes—demonstrates balance at the biological level, which is according to divine orchestration. The balance evident in all of creation points to a purposeful, intelligent design imbued with heavenly love and care. Through this lens, God is seen not only as the Creator but also as the Sustainer, ensuring that all aspects of life coexist in a beautiful, interdependent equilibrium. While it seems somewhat counterintuitive, you don't want divine energy constantly flowing at full force. Instead, we want it to flow at the optimum rate to promote life and healing. This equilibrium must also include balancing divine energy and placing it in a state of coherence that aligns with divine laws.

The idea that biophotons could be manifestations of divine energy is rooted in various spiritual and esoteric traditions. Many believe that biophotons represent a tangible connection between the human body and the divine realm. Some arguments for this theory include:

Sacred geometry. Sacred geometry is the belief that certain geometric shapes and patterns have spiritual significance. These shapes are often found in nature, art, and architecture and are thought to represent the underlying order of the universe. A circle symbolizes wholeness, infinity, and the cyclical nature of life. The square symbolizes stability and a protective boundary that shields us from negative influences. The triangle symbolizes the divine, spiritual connection, and the unification of the mind, body, and spirit. Biophotons have been shown to be involved in the organization and structure of biological systems, mirroring the principles of sacred geometry found in many spiritual traditions. This suggests a deep connection between the divine blueprint and the physical world.

Consciousness and intention. One theory suggests that biophotons could be involved in the intricate communication networks within the brain, including both conscious and subconscious thoughts. These photons could potentially facilitate rapid information transfer between neurons, contributing to cognitive processes and conscious experience.

Biophotons are believed to be influenced by consciousness and intention, which aligns with many spiritual beliefs about the power of thought and prayer. This raises questions about whether biophotons could be harnessed as a means of accessing higher states of consciousness or even communicating with the divine.

Energetic resonance. Energetic resonance suggests that our thoughts and feelings, which are forms of energy, can vibrate at specific frequencies. These vibrations can influence our physical and emotional well-being, as well as our conscious and subconscious thoughts. When we consciously focus on a thought or emotion, we are essentially tuning into a specific frequency. This frequency can then attract similar vibrations, both within us and in our external environment. Our subconscious mind is continuously processing information and forming beliefs. These beliefs, frequently formed from past experiences and conditioning, can also vibrate at specific frequencies. Biophotons operate at extremely low frequencies, which are thought to be within the range of subtle energies often associated with spiritual practices such as meditation and prayer. This resonance could provide a mechanism for connecting with divine energy.

Quantum entanglement. Quantum entanglement is a fascinating phenomenon where two particles become interconnected, regardless of distance. When one particle's state changes, the other instantaneously changes as well. This instantaneous connection has led some to speculate about its potential connection to divine energy and healing. Biophotons have been shown to exhibit quantum entanglement properties, which suggests that they can become connected and influence each other across vast distances. Practices such as prayer and visualization may harness the power of quantum entanglement to bring about positive changes in our physical and emotional health. The idea of connecting to God through quantum entanglement is fascinating and powerful.

Biophotons may play a role in cellular communication, allowing cells to exchange information and coordinate responses to stress, injury, or infection. They may also influence key biological processes, such as gene expression, enzyme activity, and metabolic functions. Through these activities, biophotons may influence biological systems and maintain, promote, or restore human health.

If biophotons are indeed manifestations of divine energy, it would have profound implications for our understanding of consciousness, human experience, and healing. An understanding of biophoton dynamics could lead to new approaches for maintaining cellular health, treating diseases, or even enhancing cognitive function. As we continue to study biophotons and their properties, we may uncover new insights into the intricate web of connections between our physical bodies, our minds, and the divine realm.

Divine Energy Is the Source of Life, Health, and Healing

The concept of divine energy as the source of life, health, and healing reverences it as the foundation to existence and health. Furthermore, it recognizes that our bodies are divinely designed to maintain a state of health and will do so if the divine energy is abundantly vigorous and active. It acknowledges that living organisms possess a vital force distinct from physical or chemical processes. It invites individuals to explore their relationship with themselves and their Creator. By recognizing the potential of divine energy in health and healing, people can deepen their connection with the ultimate source of healing.

In the intricate interplay between science and spirituality, the concept of divine energy offers a profound lens through which we can view the mysteries of life, health, and healing. It reminds us that the essence of existence transcends what is currently measurable, pointing to a sacred force that underlies all creation. Whether through faith, prayer, or the subtle emissions of biophotons, we catch glimpses of a divine mechanism at work, harmonizing the physical and spiritual realms. This perspective calls us to honor the divine spark within us, fostering a deeper connection with our Creator and the miraculous design of our bodies. By embracing the potential of divine energy, we not only cultivate physical healing but also nurture our spiritual well-being, aligning ourselves with the eternal source of life and light.

Soundwaves and Brain Function

Certain soundwaves influence brain function, perception of time and space, and spiritual experiences by altering brainwave activity, stimulating consciousness, and potentially tuning the brain to higher states of awareness. These effects may relate to connecting with the Divine and harnessing the healing energy of the universe.

Soundwaves interact with the brain through entrainment, where external frequencies synchronize brain activity. Different frequencies correspond to different states of consciousness:

- Theta & Delta Waves (4-0.5 Hz). Many people report timelessness, astral experiences, and divine encounters in these states.
- Schumann Resonance. Some claim that tuning into the Earth's natural frequency can synchronize human consciousness with nature and enhance spiritual awareness.

When specific frequencies are played (via binaural beats, solfeggio tones, or resonance therapy), they can shift consciousness into altered states, allowing for deeper perception.

By using soundwaves to enter meditative states, the body can tap into universal energy for healing. Brainwave entrainment helps restore neurological balance and reduce stress. Solfeggio frequencies are believed to repair DNA and harmonize the body. Sacred sounds (mantras, chants, or Tibetan bowls) may align energy fields, enhancing self-healing abilities.

CHAPTER FIVE

The Divine Interconnectedness Between All Life

A profound interconnectedness exists between all forms of life. They are collectively part of a unified whole emanating from a fundamental divine energy. Humans, animals, and plants are expressions of this energy. As a result, they share essential qualities and relationships that enable them to support each other. Many cultures throughout history have recognized and celebrated this interconnectedness, often embedding it in their spiritual beliefs and practices. Indigenous cultures, for instance, view the land, water, and all living beings as sacred and interconnected, emphasizing a deep respect for nature and an understanding that the health of one component affects the well-being of all. Similarly, many indigenous tribes embody this interconnectedness in their storytelling and rituals, teaching lessons about the balance of ecosystems and the vital role each species plays. By honoring this intrinsic connection, these cultures promote a universal worldview that fosters sustainability, community, and reverence for the natural world, ultimately inspiring us to cultivate similar respect and responsibility in our contemporary society.

Unity in Diversity: Embracing the Interconnectedness of Life and Divine Energy for Healing

This profound interconnectedness suggests that all forms of life are woven together in a delicate tapestry of existence, where each thread plays a vital role in sustaining the whole. At the core of this unity is the recognition that all living beings are manifestations of a shared divine energy, which fosters a sense of kinship and mutual dependence among them. Humans, as conscious stewards of the Earth, have a unique responsibility to cultivate harmony and balance within this interconnected web. Animals contribute to ecosystems through their roles as pollinators, predators, and prey, while plants perform the vital task of producing oxygen and food through photosynthesis. This intricate relationship is further deepened by the ways in which life forms communicate and interact—be it through symbiotic partnerships, such as those seen in the mutualistic relationships between bees and flowers, or through the more subtle exchanges of emotions and reactions observed in families and communities. Recognizing this essential interconnectedness encourages a holistic understanding of our place in the universe, prompting humans to embrace stewardship, compassion, and respect for all living beings. This perspective not only enriches our relationship with nature but also deepens our spiritual awareness, inviting us to engage with the world around us as a harmonious part of a greater whole, united by a divine source that flows through all living things.

Since other naturally occurring things were created with divine energy, they are saturated with and fueled by it and therefore work harmoniously with organic systems created by the same energy. Plants and other organic materials have evolved alongside humans over millennia. This close relationship means that the biochemical compounds found in these organisms are often compatible with human physiology. Through this complex connectedness of all living things, a synergy of energies is formed. This divine energy can be thought of as a life force that interacts positively with the human body's energy systems, enhancing vitality and promoting healing. This means that natural solutions from plants and other organic materials are not only compatible with but also preferred for healing the human body.

The notion that naturally occurring things are created with divine energy, sustaining the organic systems derived from the same source, greatly shapes our understanding of health and healing. Incorporating practices like aromatherapy, natural supplements, and energy healing therapies can facilitate alignment with divine energy, augmenting the body's ability to heal. By recognizing the inherent connection between divine energy, nature, and human well-being, individuals and practitioners can cultivate approaches that align with these natural principles, ultimately fostering health, balance, and harmony.

The Transformative Role of Faith and Hope in Healing

To identify natural solutions that harness divine energy for healing, those that affect biophoton emission, influence the human biofield, change vibrational frequency, enhance neuroplasticity or improve brainwave patterns, or promote physiological coherence—as measured by improved heart rate variability—will be shared.

The first step in harnessing divine energy is to believe or have hope. This exercises faith, which is a required action to harness divine energy. Hope and faith are deeply intertwined concepts, often feeding into and reinforcing one another. Hope is a precursor to faith because it represents the desire or expectation for something positive to happen or for a particular outcome to be realized, even in the face of uncertainty. It is the initial spark that motivates individuals to believe in possibilities beyond their current reality. When we hope for change, healing, or fulfillment, we open ourselves to the idea that there is something beyond our present circumstances, which can lead us to develop faith.

Conversely, faith acts as a bolster to hope. When individuals cultivate faith—belief in something greater, a higher purpose, or a positive outcome—it can enhance their sense of hope, making it more robust and resilient. This faith provides assurance and context to the hopes we hold, transforming them into something more substantial. When people experience the fruits of their faith, they often find their hopes are validated, creating a cycle where their hopeful outlook reinforces their beliefs and convictions.

As one navigates through life's challenges and experiences instances where hope bears fruit through faith, the relationship between the two becomes cyclical. Strengthening one enhances the other, creating a positive feedback loop: hope inspires faith, which in turn revitalizes hope. This dynamic interplay encourages resilience, allowing individuals to maintain their aspirations and convictions even amidst adversity. Ultimately, the cyclical nature of hope and faith fosters a deeper connection to one's beliefs and desires, illustrating how they can work hand in hand to guide and uplift individuals throughout their journeys.

The power of belief in healing is a fascinating topic that has been explored for centuries. While the exact mechanisms of how hope and faith unite us with divine energy are not fully understood, numerous studies suggest a strong connection between positive thinking, faith, and improved health outcomes. Research indicates that individuals who maintain a hopeful outlook and believe in their ability to heal are often more motivated to adhere to treatment plans, manage stress, and engage in healthy behaviors. Furthermore, practices such as prayer, meditation, and mindfulness can enhance emotional well-being, further contributing to physical health. This interplay between mental and physical health focuses us on the importance of addressing the psychological aspects of healing, reinforcing the notion that belief itself can be a potent catalyst for recovery and resilience.

The placebo effect was discussed earlier, but it warrants further discussion here. This well-documented phenomenon demonstrates the power of the mind to influence the body. When a person believes a treatment will be effective, their body may respond positively, even if the treatment is an inactive placebo. Despite no active substance being administered, the placebo effect harnesses the true source of healing, divine energy, which triggers physiological and psychological benefits.

Essentially, when you believe you are receiving an effective treatment, your brain triggers responses consistent with the desired and expected effects of the intervention. Brain imaging studies show that placebo treatments activate specific brain regions associated with pain relief, emotional regulation, and reward.[44,45] Engaging in belief or faith in a treatment can connect individuals to divine energy and lead to neuroplastic changes in the brain. Neuroplasticity is the brain's ability to reorganize itself by forming new neural connections throughout life. It plays a crucial role in physical healing by facilitating recovery and adaptation after injuries, illnesses, or chronic conditions. This adaptability enables the brain to compensate for damage and helps restore lost functions, enhance motor skills, and manage pain.

The Nexus of Neuroplasticity and Divine Energy

While the connection between neuroplasticity and divine energy may not be directly established in scientific literature, there are intriguing intersections between the two concepts, particularly in the context of mental, emotional, and spiritual healing. Many holistic and energy healing practices emphasize relaxation, which can create an optimal environment for neuroplasticity to occur. Neuroplasticity plays a crucial role in trauma recovery, allowing individuals to rewire negative thought patterns and emotional responses. Practices that involve divine energy or healing can facilitate this process by helping individuals access deeper emotional states, enhancing the healing experience. While more empirical research is necessary to establish direct correlations between neuroplasticity and divine energy, the connections between mental states, emotional healing, and brain function highlight that they may mutually reinforce each other in the pursuit of well-being and healing.

Despite being only two percent of the average human's body weight, the brain consumes a disproportionate twenty percent of the body's energy. This energy, primarily in the form of glucose, is essential for the brain's complex functions, including neural signaling, synaptic plasticity, and cognitive functions. Glucose is the brain's preferred energy source. It's transported across the blood-brain barrier and utilized by neurons to produce ATP. Compelling research suggests that disruptions in this energy metabolism can lead to various neurological disorders, such as Alzheimer's disease, Parkinson's disease, and stroke..[46,47,48,49] Energy metabolism efficiency in the brain is directly influenced by molecules like brain-derived neurotrophic factor (BDNF) and insulin-like growth factor 1, which regulate both energy balance and neuronal plasticity. To optimize brain health, it is essential to support energy metabolism, or the flow of divine energy in the brain.

Neuroplasticity can be measured molecularly (blood samples evaluating BDNF, BDNF levels in cerebrospinal fluid, and quantifying BDNF mRNA levels through gene expression studies), structural imaging (MRI or cortical thickness volume), functional imaging (fMRI; positron emission tomography, or PET), electrophysical techniques (transcranial magnetic stimulation, paired associative stimulation, EEG), neurochemical techniques (magnetic resonance spectroscopy), or behavioral and cognitive testing (improvement in motor skills, memory, or problem-solving abilities). By leveraging neuroplasticity, physical healing becomes a dynamic process where the brain adapts, compensates, and reconfigures itself to overcome challenges and restore function, emphasizing the interrelation between the nervous system and overall health.

The prefrontal cortex plays a role in the mind-body relationship, enabling individuals to bridge their thoughts and emotions with physical health. Interestingly, if prefrontal functioning of the brain is impaired, the placebo effect is significantly diminished or absent altogether. The prefrontal cortex, located at the front of the brain, is responsible for various higher-order cognitive functions, including decision-making, emotional regulation, self-awareness, social behavior, and impulse control. The prefrontal cortex plays a crucial role in regulating emotions, which is essential for mental and emotional well-being. When individuals connect with divine energy—whether through meditation, prayer, or other spiritual practices—they often experience improved emotional health. This connection may help optimize the function of the prefrontal cortex, enhancing its ability to manage stress and negative emotions. The prefrontal cortex is integral to making decisions and processing information. When people seek divine energy or engage in spiritual practices, they may cultivate a greater sense of intuition and insight. This heightened awareness can lead to improved access to divine energy. The prefrontal cortex synthesizes information from various brain regions, allowing individuals to reflect on their experiences and learn from them. This process is important in understanding personal health journeys and making informed choices that resonate with the principles of natural healing and connection to divine energy.

Some theories propose that the prefrontal cortex's function is integral to experiences of transcendence and spiritual connection. This suggests that activities like meditation promote neurochemical changes that facilitate experiences of divine energy—potentially leading to profound effects on well-being and health. By engaging the prefrontal cortex through mindfulness, intention, prayer, gratitude, and self-reflection, individuals can amplify their connection to divine energy, enriching their healing processes and overall well-being. This relationship between neuroscience and spirituality underscores the holistic nature of health, illustrating the powerful ways in which our mental, emotional, and spiritual dimensions can contribute to healing.

Exploring the Frequencies of Healing and Cellular Vibrations

It is possible that divine energy can be measured by frequency, which is the number of times a sine wave repeats, or completes, a positive-to-negative cycle. Imagine a swing. When you push it, it swings back and forth. Each time it swings from one side to the other, that's one cycle. How fast it swings back and forth is its frequency. Electricity works in a similar way. It flows back and forth, creating a cycle. The number of times it flows back and forth in a second is its frequency. This is measured in Hertz (Hz). For example, if electricity flows back and forth sixty times in a second, we say it has a frequency of 60 Hertz. This is the standard frequency for most homes and businesses in North America, while other parts of the world, like Europe and Asia, often use a 50 Hz standard.

The concepts of vibrational frequency and healing, particularly in the context of cells and human beings, are rooted in both scientific principles and holistic health practices. The premise is that everything in the universe, including human cells and the human body, vibrates at specific frequencies.[50] Indeed, emerging research suggests that cellular vibration patterns can distinguish health cells from diseased cells..[51] Specifically, the researchers observed that the membranes of cancerous cells displayed larger amplitudes (a measure of the wave's intensity and strength) of less correlated (less synchronized or coordinated) surface vibrations and were softer when compared to their corresponding healthy cells. Understanding these frequencies and vibrational patterns can provide insights into health, healing, and the potential to reverse destructive energy patterns associated with illness.

At a fundamental level, all matter, including human cells, is composed of atoms and molecules that are in constant motion, vibrating at specific frequencies. This motion occurs within a range of energies and wavelengths, which can be measured and analyzed. Different frequencies, amplitudes, and correlations are thought to correspond to different states of health and well-being. For instance, healthy cells vibrate at higher frequencies, while diseased or unhealthy cells may vibrate at lower frequencies. Bruce Tainio, a researcher and developer of the world's first frequency monitor, found that a healthy human body resonates at a frequency of 62 to 70 MHz; and dropping to 58 MHz or below initiates the disease process..[52] Everything we do—food and drink we consume, thoughts we have, sleep we get, how much we move, and much more—either helps maintain this healthy frequency or reduces it.

In *Energy Medicine: The Scientific Basis*, Dr. James Oschman explores the concept that human cells operate within specific frequency ranges and possess the ability to resonate with subtle energy fields both within the body and in the surrounding environment. He presents a detailed analysis of how cellular communication and function can be influenced by these energy patterns. Oschman integrates findings from various scientific disciplines, including biology and physics, to illustrate how energy fields play a crucial role in health and healing processes. He argues that understanding these energy dynamics can provide valuable insights into the mechanisms of alternative therapies and enhance conventional medical practices. Overall, his work emphasizes the significance of energy in both the physiological and energetic aspects of human health, advocating for a more integrative approach to medicine that acknowledges the interplay between energy fields and biological systems.

Human emotions carry vibrational frequencies. They aren't measured exactly like body energy is through electromagnetic activity. Instead, the frequency of emotions is linked to physiological changes in brainwaves, heart coherence, and electromagnetic activity. Emotions fundamentally influence bodily frequencies by altering their bioelectrical patterns in the body. Positive emotions (such as love, joy, and gratitude) resonate at higher frequencies, while negative emotions (such as fear, anger, and resentment) resonate at lower frequencies..[53] The more powerful the positive emotion, the higher the vibrational frequency. For example, emotions like contentment and acceptance typically vibrate between 250 to 310 Hz, while joy, love, and gratitude are even higher, vibrating above 500 Hz. Contrarily, negative emotions tend to vibrate below 100 Hz. And these emotions don't just influence your frequency for the time that you feel them, emotions can be stored in your cells continually acting as electromagnetic energy that positively or negatively influences your well-being. Higher frequencies correspond to higher energy levels, while lower frequencies are associated with lower energy levels.

Bacteria, fungi, and viruses vibrate at their own frequency and this influences human frequency. Environmental pollutants, chemicals in food, and heavy metals can disrupt cellular vibrations. Chronic exposure to these harmful frequencies can culminate in various health issues, including immune dysfunction, inflammation, chronic pain, and even chronic diseases like cancer and autoimmunity.

Each type of cell in the body has a unique vibrational frequency, which is influenced by various internal and external factors, including emotional states, environmental stressors, and nutritional inputs. The frequency of the cells that make up your brain produces a different "song" than the sound of the cells of your heart. Healthy cellular function is dependent on maintaining optimal vibrational frequencies, or the cycling of divine energy. Evidence suggests that certain frequencies can repel disease, while other frequencies destroy disease. When cells, organs, or tissues function poorly or become diseased, they no longer produce the optimal resonant frequency (sound) to maintain health.

Beyond the Limits of Science: Unveiling the Miracles of Faith and Divine Intervention

Just like the Bible, modern history is full of individuals who experienced unbelievable healing through divine petitions. One such example is an elderly woman from South Africa diagnosed with stage 4 terminal cancer.[54] Christian missionaries found her in a care center for the elderly and noted that she was full of faith in God and believed He would, not could, heal her. Her breast cancer had spread throughout her entire body and her prognosis was not good. The Christian missionaries prayed with and for her, each exercising faith that she would be healed. Incredibly, the day after these prayers of faith, the Christian missionaries got a call that this woman's tumor had inexplicably disappeared.

Similarly, what can only be described as a divine intervention occurred in Spanish Fork, Utah, leading to saving a precious infant's life..[55] A baby survived nearly fourteen hours in a car that crashed into a frigid Utah river. The baby's mother, Lynn Jennifer Groesbeck, lost control of her car, striking a cement barrier and plunging into the river. While Lynn did not survive, her 18-month-old daughter Lily did because first responders on the scene were guided by an adult voice from inside the car pleading, "Help me, help me." Following the voice, three firefighters and two police officers rushed into the river and found Lily hanging upside down in her car seat just above the frigid water. How is this possible when Lynn was reportedly killed on impact?

Another woman received a second chance on life after she was revived from a heart attack after being declared clinically dead for forty-five minutes..[56] Kathy Patten had a heart attack after arriving at the hospital to support her daughter who was giving birth. CPR was started when her pulse was lost, and after nearly an hour of resuscitation efforts, she was revived. One could argue that two miracles occurred in this story. First, she happened to have the heart attack while in a hospital, where she could receive appropriate rescue healthcare. And second, she was brought back to life through extraordinary efforts after almost an hour of being clinically dead.

Just because these miraculous healings can't be explained doesn't mean they didn't happen. You cannot deny the experiences of others simply because they can't be explained. In fact, science can't truly explain; it can only observe what we currently know. This fact was emphasized by the fourth and fifth-century theologian and philosopher Saint Augustine, also known as Augustine of Hippo, when he reportedly said, "Miracles are not contrary to nature, but only contrary to what we know about nature." Frankly, science has severe limitations. One of its greatest limitations is that it relies upon observation of our environment by the limited tools we have for observing that environment. Science, therefore, is not absolute because it is only substantiated by the most supported interpretation of scientific observation, the scientific premise with the least opposition to that viewpoint. In other words, science can only observe things within the scope of its limitations, not the potential of experiences beyond this. As humans, we need to take a more open-minded approach that considers the possibility of phenomena beyond the realm of current scientific understanding. Countless other stories just like this could be shared, but suffice it so say miracles have, are, and will continue to happen.

The reality is that we live in an infinite universe and have a very limited understanding of what resides in that universe, let alone how everything works. We can't observe, yet alone explain, everything that influences and shapes mankind, including unseen energy. Do we really understand how the central nervous system works? Not even close. We understand very little based on our incomplete observation capabilities. Since we cannot observe all things, we cannot disregard that forces beyond our observation, and natural laws beyond our understanding, are influencing our conclusions.

An overreliance on science, or scientism, excludes the one absolute source of Truth—Almighty God. Absolute Truth is not swayed by public opinion, popularity, or economic and political agendas. Unfortunately, too many people victimize themselves anew when they find out they have been bamboozled by manufactured "truth" because they refuse to seek the actual Truth. Faith and belief can offer a complementary perspective to scientific inquiry, providing a sense of meaning and purpose in the face of uncertainty.

Embracing Faith, Suffering, and Divine Timing

While not every person who petitions God for healing, will receive it, some do. Many people wonder if they lacked sufficient faith, if they did something wrong, or if God simply doesn't love them as much as He loves others, when healing doesn't occur. Why this discrepancy? David A. Bednar answered this question in this way: "Even if we have strong faith, many mountains will not be moved. And not all of the sick and infirm will be healed. If all opposition were curtailed, if all maladies were removed, then the primary purposes of the Father's plan would be frustrated. Many of the lessons we are to learn in mortality can be received only through the things we experience and sometimes suffer. And God expects and trusts us to face temporary mortal adversity with His help so we can learn what we need to learn and ultimately become what we are to become in eternity." In other words, we need to accept the Lord's will and timing and realize that His timing may not be until we are released from mortality. There is a divine plan or reason for everything, including suffering and healing. His plan is always greater than ours. Even when divine help is sought, there are many factors at play that can affect the outcome. For those who feel unhealed, exploring these various dimensions may provide insights and lead to new paths of understanding and growth.

Aligning Ourselves with the Divine Rhythm That Sustains Life

In the intricate tapestry of existence, the divine interconnectedness between all life reveals itself as both profound and humbling. Every being, every element, every moment is part of a symphony where the individual notes merge into a greater melody. This interdependence teaches us that our choices ripple far beyond our immediate perception, influencing the vast web of life in ways we may never fully understand. The Creator's divine energy creates a network of connections that transcends physical boundaries. By embracing this truth, we honor the sacred bond that unites us with Him, the Earth, its creatures, and each other—a bond that calls us to live with reverence, compassion, and purpose. In recognizing our shared essence, we awaken to the divine harmony that weaves us into one universal whole and align ourselves with the divine rhythm that sustains all life.

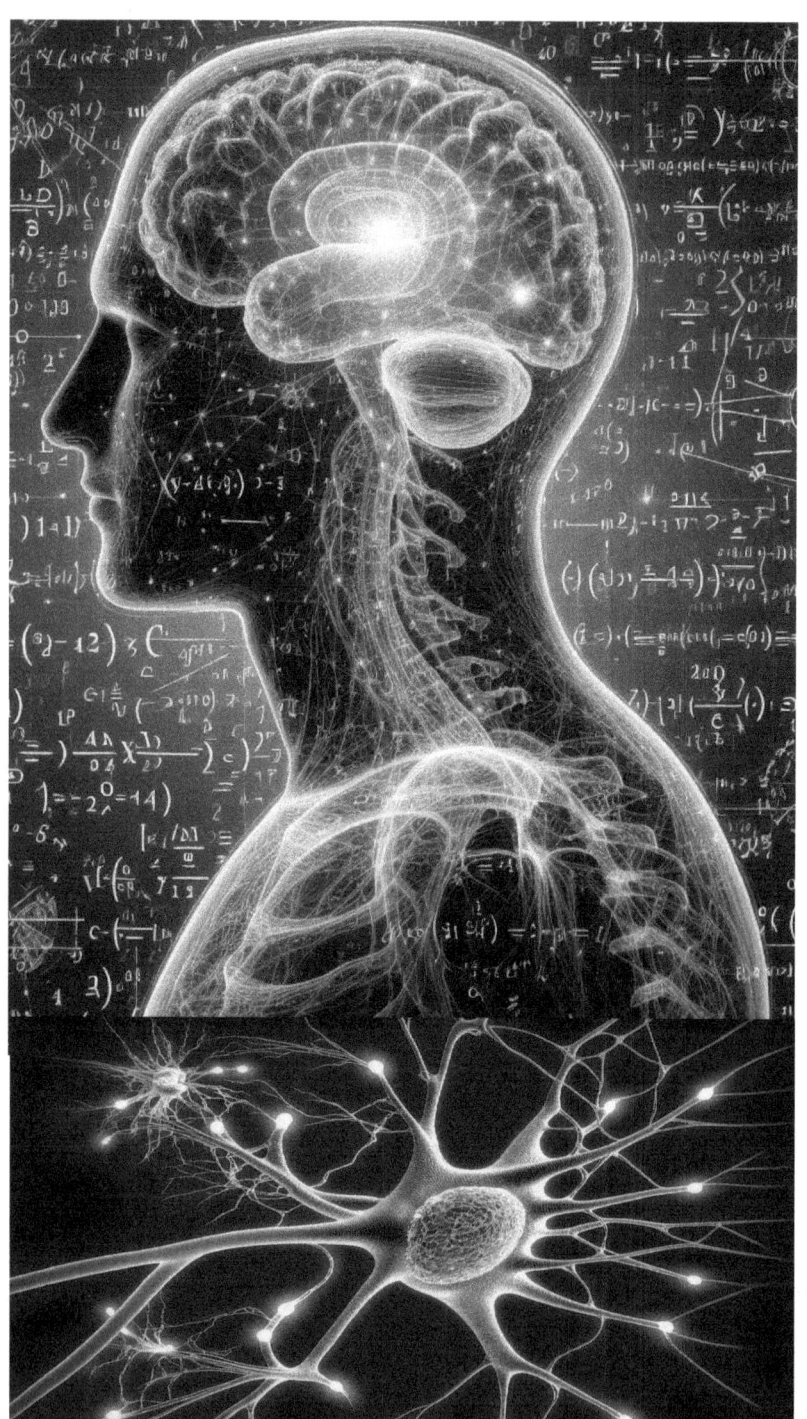

CHAPTER SIX

Lifestyle Behaviors that Harness Divine Energy: Nutrition, Physical Activity, and Relaxation Techniques

You have made it through the intense science and deep philosophy of divine energy, and you're now ready to learn how to wield it for healing purposes. There are a few important factors that must be considered for peak divine energy flow and optimal healing. The first step is identifying the root cause of your health challenge, which is most likely a past emotional or spiritual experience.

Releasing Underlying Emotional and Spiritual Issues

Underlying emotional and spiritual issues must be addressed first because they disrupt the healing potential of divine energy. Remember that emotion (the heart) usually trumps logic (the brain), so issues of the heart should be prioritized. Think back to when your challenge started. Was there a distressing or traumatic experience that preceded it? Do you have an unresolved unconscious belief that formed during early childhood as a result of an upsetting experience? Do you have a tragic or painful family history that could have passed on ancestral gene expression that is contributing to your current challenge? Deep-seated, often unconscious beliefs can manifest as emotional stress and, in turn, contribute to emotional, mental, or physical health problems.

Your healing process requires bringing awareness to and identifying past emotional and spiritual experiences that are contributing to your current health concern. Once you've identified the most likely emotional or spiritual cause, focus on the feelings and beliefs surrounding this event. The goal is to recalibrate these beliefs to unblock divine energy and promote healing. By addressing these unconscious memories, you are freeing your cells from a burden that is disrupting their function.

Reframing Thoughts and Beliefs Through Truth Declarations

Truth declarations replace negative, limiting beliefs or thoughts that can hinder emotional and physical well-being. They are designed to align one's mindset with healing principles and foster a positive and empowering outlook. Your truth statement should be tailored to your individual experiences and beliefs and resonate with you personally. It should be crafted in a positive, affirmative manner so that it can reinforce positive thoughts and beliefs, counteracting any negative self-perceptions. Truth declarations work best when they emphasize themes of love, healing, worthiness, and acceptance. Here are a few examples of powerful truth declarations:

> *"I am worthy of love and healing. My body is skillful in healing itself through divine energy."*
>
> *"Every cell in my body radiates health and vitality; loving and healing memories are permeating my cells."*
>
> *"I am experiencing healing on all levels as I am surrounded by the love of God."*
>
> *"I forgive myself for past mistakes, and I release any guilt or shame, freeing myself from the burdens of the past."*

Truth declarations serve as powerful tools for transformation, enabling individuals to reframe their thoughts and beliefs in a way that promotes healing and well-being.

Prayer: The Channel Through Which Divine Energy Is Accessed

Prayer should be central to your healing process no matter what means or methods you choose to stimulate the healing effects of divine energy. Since the gift of healing and the power by which all things were created comes through God, we must petition Him who is the source of life. Prayer involves setting intentions for healing, which can harness mental and emotional energies to promote well-being. Be sincere and as specific as possible in your prayers. If depression is your primary challenge, you might pray something like this:

> *I ask Thee to reveal all known and unknown thoughts, beliefs, damaging cellular memories, generational distress, and physical issues related to depression [or your specific issue] and that they be healed through the Light of Christ and Thy divine healing power. I also pray that the proficiency of Thy divine energy be amplified in me to produce maximum results.*

Prayer serves as a channel through which individuals can access divine energy, invoking it for healing purposes, whether for themselves or others.

Divine Energy Capacity Reflects Lifestyle

The question we should ask ourselves each day is "How are my daily habits surrounding nutrition, movement, sleep, stress management, smart supplementation, etc. influencing the coherence of my bodily systems?" When searching for lifestyle behaviors, natural solutions, or energy and sound healing modalities to harness the healing influence of divine energy, we can infer their effects from potential measurements of divine energy, including biophoton emission, HRV, galvanic skin response, human biofield, vibrational frequency, and neuroplasticity (or increased BDNF). Personal introspection on our own daily choices can push us toward a path fostering the body's innate ability to maintain harmony with divine energy and sustain homeostasis.

Nourishing Your Cells: The Essential Role of Nutrient-Dense Foods in Health and Energy

The foundation of your health is nutrition. Your body craves nutrients required for cellular and organ function, not calories. Focusing on calorie counting instead of nutrient quality is a misleading concept. This approach oversimplifies nutrition and shifts the emphasis to less important matters. Vitamins, minerals, and antioxidants are essential for energy production, immune function, and overall health but do not directly correlate with calories. Put simply, not all calories are the same. Indeed, promoting calorie-focused diets drives sales of low-calorie highly processed foods, meal plans, and tracking apps that line food companies' pockets with profits without improving health outcomes.

Some macronutrients—proteins, carbohydrates, and fats—are metabolized differently than other nutrients. Protein requires more energy to digest—called the thermogenic effect (TEF)—when compared to fats and carbohydrates and supports muscle building. This means that it takes more energy (calories) to digest, absorb, and metabolize protein. Studies suggest that TEF for protein can be around 20–30% of the calories consumed, compared to only 5–10% for carbohydrates and 0-3% for fats..[57] Because of this higher energy expenditure, some argue that the net caloric gain from protein is lower than its actual calorie count. Unlike fats and carbohydrates, protein is not stored in the body to a significant extent; instead, it is used to build and repair tissues or converted to energy when necessary. This means that excessive protein intake may be less likely to lead to fat accumulation compared to excess carbohydrates or fats. The body continuously uses protein for various metabolic processes. Thus, its role in maintaining bodily functions may justify a different consideration of its caloric contribution.

You must fuel your body with nutrient-dense foods. By fueling your body with these foods, you are providing it with the building blocks it needs for immune health, brain function, cellular repair, energy production, and overall well-being. Fueling your body intentionally develops a greater sense of connection to your body and will also influence divine energy by generating ATP. ATP provides the energy necessary for various cellular processes, including muscle contraction, neurotransmission, and cellular repair. Healthy cells rely on adequate ATP production to function optimally, which is essential for maintaining physical health. An abundance of ATP promotes effective healing processes in the body. Essentially, providing your body with the fuel it needs to efficiently produce ATP, safeguards your supply of divine energy for healthy cellular processes and healing to work optimally.

One way to eat the best food for your body is to base it on nutrigenomics. Nutrigenomics is the study of how our genes and gene expression are influenced by different nutrients and dietary patterns. This field combines aspects of nutrition and genomics to provide personalized dietary recommendations that can promote optimal health. Genetic variations can affect how individuals metabolize nutrients. For example, some people may have genetic variants that influence their ability to absorb certain vitamins or minerals, such as vitamin D or folate. Nutrigenomics can identify these pathways and offer tailored supplementation or food sources. By analyzing an individual's genetic profile, nutrigenomics can help identify specific nutrient needs and sensitivities. This means that dietary recommendations can be tailored to optimize health based on an individual's genetic makeup, making nutrition more effective for health improvement and disease prevention. Without nutrigenomics, you are stuck with experimentation through trial and error to see what diet suits you most.

There are various nutrigenomics tests available that analyze different aspects of your genetics in relation to nutrition. You can obtain nutrigenomics tests through several platforms:

- Direct-to-consumer genetic testing companies
- Health and wellness clinics
- Nutritionists or dieticians
- Laboratories offering genetic testing

Emerging research demonstrates that various aspects of nutrition benefit HRV, both immediately and in the longer term.[58] The Mediterranean diet is a healthy eating pattern inspired by the traditional diets of countries bordering the Mediterranean Sea, rich in fruits, vegetables, whole grains, legumes, nuts, and seeds. Healthy fats, primarily from olive oil, are incorporated, while lean protein sources like fish, poultry, and legumes are favored over red meat. Dairy products are consumed in moderation, and red wine may be enjoyed in small amounts. This diet promotes a lifestyle that includes regular physical activity and stress management, contributing to overall health and well-being.

Using a food-frequency questionnaire to establish how closely middle-aged male twins adhered to the Mediterranean diet, it was observed that the Mediterranean diet increases HRV.[59] This suggests that this pattern of eating can improve physiological resilience and health, indicating enhanced utilization of divine energy. While it is difficult to assign these benefits to one aspect of the Mediterranean diet, other research implies that consuming omega-3 fatty acids affects ion channels and calcium-regulatory proteins..[60] Fatty acids are incorporated into the cell membrane, leading to changes in cardiac electrical activity and HRV increases. This indicates HRV improvements are a result of the body's built-in pacemaker and resulting electrical impulses, rather than regulation by the autonomic nervous system. These findings highlight the profound connection between dietary choices and the body's intrinsic mechanisms for harnessing and optimizing divine energy for improved health and resilience.

The concept of "high vibrational foods" (e.g., dark leafy greens, blueberries, mangoes, garlic, cinnamon, dates, and fermented foods) refers to foods that are believed to carry a high level of energy and life force, and proponents of this idea suggest that consuming such foods can positively influence a person's vibrational frequency. Some research even explores the idea that living foods emit biophotons..[61] This area of study suggests that the vibrational properties of foods might be linked to their freshness and natural state. While the scientific basis for measuring vibrational frequency in foods and its direct effects on human physiology is limited, there are some areas of research that indirectly support the idea that nutrition can influence divine energy and possibly even the perceived vibrational state of individuals.

High-vibrational foods typically include raw fruits, vegetables, nuts, seeds, and whole grains. These foods are rich in vitamins, minerals, and phytonutrients, which can support overall health, vitality, and energy levels. High-vibrational foods tend to be less processed and more natural. The idea is that the more of these foods you eat, the greater your vibrational frequency and health.

An argument could be made that the genetic modification and selective breeding of crops have misaligned them from their divine blueprint and even diminished the divine energy they contain. Genetically modified organisms (GMOs) are viewed as unnatural because they involve human intervention at a fundamental biological level. Altering the genetic structure of a plant through modification or selective breeding may be seen as disrupting its original design, potentially leading to crops that lack the intended vitality, nutritional value, or spiritual essence. Modifications in the genetic makeup of plants can have cascading effects on ecosystems. The introduction of GMOs might disrupt local biodiversity, which some may argue is an essential component of the natural order and balance created by a divine source. The consequences of genetic modifications can be unpredictable, potentially leading to ecological or health-related issues that are violations of natural and divine laws.

BDNF is most active in areas of the brain involved in cognition, namely the hippocampus and cerebral cortex. Essential for the maintenance, survival, growth, and differentiation of neurons, BDNF stimulates neuroplasticity to enhance learning capacity and memory formation. Polyphenols—a class of compounds found abundantly in plant foods—are linked with improved brain health. For example, polyphenols found in green tea (EGCG), turmeric (curcumin), grapes (resveratrol), and cocoa (cocoa flavanols) are strongly associated with higher cognitive function, improved mood, and protection against various brain diseases.[62] While significant emphasis is placed on the antioxidant properties of polyphenols, they can improve brain health by regulating specific cellular signaling pathways (cAMP-response element-binding protein) that impact genes that express BDNF.[63] By activating this pathway and increasing BDNF levels, polyphenols improve divine energy flow in the brain and subsequently enhance overall brain health and resilience.

Less commonly used in Western societies, rye bread offers more nutritional benefits than white bread. It also significantly increases BDNF in comparison to white bread. A randomized crossover study compared the effects of consuming rye kernel-based bread (RKB) or a white wheat flour-based bread (WWB) in healthy young adults.[64] BDNF concentrations were investigated in the morning after fasting for 10.5 hours after consuming the bread the night before, and after three consecutive evening meals with RKB and WWB. The RKB evening meal increased BDNF concentrations by 27 percent. Since WWB is a processed food that has much of its nutrition stripped during processing, it makes sense that a more whole food would maintain greater divine energy and consequently have a bigger impact on BDNF. The researchers concluded that rye is beneficial to neuronal integrity and cognitive functions, possibly due to its fermentation in the gut, which leads to the production of beneficial short-chain fatty acids.

Another comparison, this time of processed cheese versus mold-fermented cheese, showed that the least processed food produced the greatest impact on BDNF.[65] Older Japanese women with mild cognitive impairment were randomized to consume 33.4 g of mold-fermented cheese or processed non-mold-fermented cheese daily for three months. After three months there was a three-month period where the participants received no cheese (washout period), followed by three months of consuming the other cheese (crossover). Although consuming the mold-fermented cheese did not translate to improved cognition according to the Mini-Mental State Examination, significant increases in BDNF levels were observed. It seems consuming foods that have undergone less processing can have a greater impact on BDNF levels, confirming the dietary recommendations of holistic practitioners to eat whole, fresh foods as much as possible.

The Vital Link: How Physical Activity Transforms Health and Energy Flow

The phrase "inactivity is the new smoking" highlights the significant health risks associated with a sedentary lifestyle. While smoking remains a major health hazard, research has increasingly shown that physical inactivity can have similarly detrimental effects on our bodies.[66] Basically, research concluded that your risk of stroke and heart attack increases 65 percent when your physical activity is poor compared to ideal, while it increases 77 percent if you smoke. Physical inactivity also increases your risk of type 2 diabetes, certain cancers, and mental health issues.[67,68,69] Regular physical activity helps boost the immune system, making it more effective at fighting off infections. Inactivity, on the other hand, can compromise immune function. Physical activity slows down the aging process by preserving muscle mass, bone density, and cognitive function. Inactivity, conversely, can accelerate aging and lead to premature decline. It's important to recognize that physical inactivity poses a significant threat to your health. Conversely, living an active lifestyle reduces your risk of illness and chronic disease, and enhances your health span.

Exercise influences biophoton emission through its effects on cellular metabolism, oxidative stress, and overall physiological activity. As a reminder, biophotons are weak emissions of light produced by living cells during biochemical reactions, particularly those involving reactive oxygen species (ROS). Exercise elevates cellular metabolism to meet increased energy demands, particularly in muscles. This heightened metabolic activity generates more ROS as byproducts of cellular respiration, which can lead to a temporary increase in biophoton emission. While some ROS can be harmful, they also play a role in cellular signaling and can contribute to biophoton emission.

Not surprisingly, intense or endurance training may exceed the capacity of the body's antioxidant defenses, creating oxidative stress. Quite the reverse, regular, moderate exercise enhances the body's antioxidant defenses over time, potentially stabilizing biophoton emissions. Exercise stimulates DNA repair and cellular health, potentially affecting the dynamics of biophoton emission. Healthier cells with optimized metabolic and repair mechanisms might emit biophotons in a more balanced manner. Studies on biophoton emission and exercise are still emerging, but measuring changes in biophoton patterns during or after physical activity could provide insights into cellular health, stress levels, and the systemic effects of exercise on the body.

The human biofield is often described as an energetic field that surrounds and interpenetrates the body, reflecting a complex interplay of biological, emotional, and spiritual dimensions. While scientific investigation of the biofield is still evolving, it is reasonable to make a connection between physical activity and its impact on the biofield. Physical activity enhances blood circulation, which enhances the distribution of oxygen and nutrients throughout the body. Improved blood flow also helps remove toxins and potentially unblock stagnant energy, allowing for a smoother flow of divine energy. Exercise also stimulates the lymphatic system, which is crucial for immune function and detoxification. This improved lymphatic flow may help maintain the integrity of the biofield by removing toxins and promoting a healthier energetic environment.

Physical activity is known to reduce stress, anxiety, and depression through the release of neurotransmitters like endorphins and serotonin. Managing stress can lead to a more balanced biofield, reducing energetic blockages caused by negative emotional states. Participating in physical activities with others can create a sense of community and belonging, which enriches one's biofield. Positive social interactions can lead to an uplifting of personal energy, fostering a supportive biofield that extends to others. Group activities may allow for the exchange of energies, creating a collective biofield where individual energetic contributions enhance the overall well-being of the participants. It may be a means whereby those with currently weaker biofields could experience strengthened biofields from those in the fitness class with stronger biofields.

Regular physical activity can promote better posture and body alignment, allowing for more efficient energy flow. Misalignments in the body can lead to blockages or distortions in the biofield, while balanced alignment helps maintain a clear and harmonious energetic state. Lastly, engaging in physical activities can lead to a deeper connection with one's body and, by extension, with one's biofield. While the concept of the biofield encompasses both physical and energetic dimensions, maintaining an active lifestyle can be viewed as a holistic approach to fostering a vibrant and balanced energetic state. Integrating regular physical activity into daily life may therefore not only promote physical health but also enhance the overall quality and integrity of one's biofield.

Another way to quantify the way that physical activity boosts divine energy is by observing changes in neuroplasticity and BDNF expression. Physical activity alters the synaptic structure and function in various brain regions, adjusts the development of the neurovascular system (promotes angiogenesis), and modifies glial activation; all of which aids neuroplasticity..[70] At a molecular level, several neurotrophic and growth factors are improved during physical activity. Among them, BDNF expression is upregulated, facilitating optimal cognitive function through improved divine energy flow.

Our bodies are designed to move, not just for physical survival, but as a conduit to enhance the flow of divine energy. Movement serves as a bridge between the physical, emotional, and spiritual realms, allowing energy to circulate more freely and restoring balance within us. Movement stimulates the flow of divine energy, which sustains life.

Harmonizing Energy Through Mindfulness and Meditation

Mindfulness and meditation can significantly influence biophoton interactions, enhancing the body's divine energy and promoting cellular communication and coherence. Coherent light is more organized and effective in facilitating communication between cells. Think of coherent light like a perfectly synchronized choir, where every singer is on the same note and timing, producing a harmonious sound. In this analogy, the choir represents communication between cells. Just as the synchronized voices create a clear and powerful melody that resonates beautifully, coherent light enables cells to communicate more effectively, creating a well-organized and efficient exchange of information. In contrast, incoherent light would be like a group of soloists singing at different times and pitches—chaotic and less effective in conveying a message. Mindfulness and meditation encourage a state of physiological coherence—a synchronized interaction between the heart, brain, and other systems. By relaxing the body and aligning body functions, biophoton release is synchronized and the efficiency of cellular communication enhanced.

Studies have observed that meditation increases the coherence of energy fields measurable through biophoton detectors.[71] Divine energy, or the coherent light source, observed during meditation helps maintain homeostasis by heightening communication and control between cells. Other research confirms that even short-term meditation can have considerable effects on brain energy metabolism.[72] Specifically, meditation seemed to be establishing divine energy coherence by stimulating the temporal areas and basal ganglia to a higher energetic state, while simultaneously diminishing the energetic state, ATP turnover, and oxidative capacity in the frontal and occipital areas of the brain. This suggests that meditation not only fosters divine energy coherence within the body but also optimizes the brain's energetic balance, enhancing its ability to support overall health and spiritual alignment.

It comes as no surprise that mindfulness meditation also improves HRV. A clinical trial evaluated the effects of Vipassana meditation on HRV in thirty-six individuals.[73] Vipassana meditation, often called "insight meditation," is a practice that helps you see things as they truly are. It involves observing your breath, bodily sensations, thoughts, and emotions without reacting or judging them. The goal is to develop self-awareness and gain a clear understanding of how your mind works. Over time, this mindfulness can lead to greater inner peace, clarity, and freedom from negative patterns. As expected, study participants showed increased well-being as their HRV increased compared to baseline. Another randomized clinical study observed changes in chronic and acute HRV while people participated in a 10-day online-based mindfulness intervention.[74] A positive control group listened to music, while a negative control group had no intervention at all. Increased acute HRV was noted during the daily practice sessions in both the meditation and music groups. The chronic effects on HRV were more pronounced in the meditation group, where participants experienced increased HRV during both the day and night, indicating higher sleep quality. Lastly, a systemic review of published literature concluded that slow breathing, something practiced in many forms of meditation, enhances autonomic nervous system, cerebral, and psychological flexibility.[75] The researchers noted increased HRV and low-frequency power as well as enhanced brain activity (increased alpha power and decreased theta power), which are both related to emotional control and psychological well-being. These findings further emphasize the profound impact mindfulness meditation has on both physiological and psychological coherence, highlighting its potential to enhance overall well-being through increased HRV and improved emotional regulation.

Lifestyle, a Vital Pathway to Harness Divine Energy

In conclusion, the lifestyle behaviors we engage in—nutrition, physical activity, and relaxation techniques—are more than just practices for physical health; they are vital pathways through which we can harness divine energy to promote healing and balance. By nourishing our bodies with wholesome, nutrient-dense foods, moving intentionally to foster vitality, and embracing practices like meditation and deep relaxation, we align ourselves with the natural rhythms of the universe. These behaviors not only support our physical well-being, but they also enhance the flow of divine energy within us, enabling our bodies to heal, regenerate, and maintain harmony. Ultimately, when we adopt these lifestyle practices with authenticity and intention, we tap into a greater source of healing power, allowing divine energy to guide us toward a state of true health and wholeness.

The Neural Highway Connecting All Living Things

The idea of a neural highway connecting all living things and consciousness aligns with both scientific and spiritual perspectives, suggesting that all life is interconnected through an energetic and informational network. This concept relates to divine energy and healing by offering a framework where consciousness, life force, and universal intelligence flow through all beings, enabling spiritual growth, communication, and well-being. If consciousness is interconnected across a universal field, then divine energy flows through this network, affecting all life.

Neuroscience has revealed that the brain's neuronal pathways communicate through electrical and biochemical signals, forming a network of perception, memory, and awareness. Spiritual traditions extend this concept beyond the brain, viewing the body and consciousness as part of a larger divine network. Scientific evidence shows that the mind's belief system can heal the body, supporting the idea that consciousness is an active force in health. The vagus nerve, known as the "wandering nerve," connects the brain, heart, and gut, influencing emotional states, meditation experiences, and divine connection.

Since all consciousness is interconnected, divine energy can be accessed by aligning one's mind, body, and spirit with this greater network. Healing—whether physical, emotional, or spiritual—may occur when individuals tap into this interconnected energy field overseen by the Divine.

CHAPTER SEVEN

Channeling Divine Energy with Energy Healing Techniques

As previously discussed, everything in the natural world is created by the same God who created us, which means that the essence (spirit) of all natural things carries the same divine energy of creation that flows through our own bodies. This interconnectedness creates a profound harmony between the natural world and the human body, allowing us to resonate with the energy and healing properties found in nature. When we turn to natural solutions, whether in the form of plants, vitamins, herbs, minerals, or other elements of the Earth, we are engaging with energies that are not foreign to us but are intimately aligned with our own divine nature. These natural remedies work in tandem with our innate healing abilities, supporting our bodies to restore balance and health in ways that are harmonious with the universal energy that sustains all life. By acknowledging the spiritual and energetic connections between us and nature, we unlock the potential for deep healing and well-being that is rooted in divine alignment.

Alignment Through Energy Healing Modalities and Biofield Therapies

A wide variety of energy healing modalities are practiced to promote healing by balancing the energy that flows through the human body. Some of the most popular include:

- Acupuncture. An ancient Chinese practice that involves inserting thin needles into specific points on the body to balance energy flow.
- Acupressure. An energy healing modality that involves applying pressure to specific points on the body, known as acupoints, to improve the body's energy pathways, or meridians.
- Reiki. A Japanese technique focused on channeling universal life energy to promote relaxation and healing.
- Massage. A hands-on technique that manipulates soft tissues to relieve tension and promote relaxation.
- Healing touch. A gentle, hands-on therapy that promotes healing and relaxation through energy exchange.
- Therapeutic touch. A noninvasive energy therapy that uses gentle touch to promote healing and relaxation.
- Pranic healing. A technique that uses energy healing to balance and harmonize the body's energy centers, known as chakras.
- Johrei. A Japanese spiritual healing practice that involves transmitting light energy to heal physical, emotional, and spiritual imbalances.
- Qigong. A Chinese practice that combines physical postures, breathing techniques, and meditation to balance energy flow.
- Energy kinesiology. A practice that bridges the gap between traditional kinesiology and energy healing, combining the scientific understanding of the body's mechanics with the belief in energy flow and balance.
- Reflexology. A technique that applies pressure to specific points on the feet, hands, or ears to send reflex responses to distant organs and tissues of the body and improve overall well-being.

- The Healing Code. A spiritual practice that proposes that unresolved emotional and spiritual issues can manifest as physical ailments and that through prayer and specific techniques, these underlying issues can be addressed to promote healing.
- Crystal Healing. The use of crystals to balance and heal the body's energy centers and promote physical, emotional, and physical well-being.

A review of various biofield therapies, or energy healing therapies, assessed the clinical effectiveness of these therapies.[76] It included clinical trials of biofield therapies for any condition, cancer, pain, cardiovascular disease, and wound healing. The review found that biofield therapies have shown promise in reducing pain, anxiety, and improving quality of life in various patient populations. However, more rigorous research is needed to establish definitive conclusions and understand the mechanisms of action. Key challenges in studying biofield therapies identified by the researchers include the diversity of techniques, the subjective nature of many outcomes, and the difficulty in controlling for placebo effects. Recommendations for future research include larger, randomized controlled trials with rigorous methodology, the exploration of biomarkers to assess the impact of biofield therapies, and the inclusion of diverse patient populations. While robust evidence may still be emerging, the body of anecdotal experiences and preliminary findings suggests that energy healing modalities hold significant potential within the realm of alternative healing. As researchers continue to explore and overcome the challenges of studying biofield therapies, the promise they offer in alleviating suffering and enhancing well-being cannot be overlooked. A commitment to rigorous inquiry and an open-minded approach may ultimately illuminate the pathways through which these therapies can contribute meaningfully to patient care and support holistic healing practices.

Of the thirty published clinical trials on pain, the preponderance of the evidence showed significant reductions in self-reported pain and clinically relevant outcome measures. The researchers proposed that the mechanism of biofield therapies to reduce pain could be either a "bottom-up" process (reduced cellular inflammation or nociceptive signaling—the process by which the body senses and responds to noxious stimuli) or a "top-down" process (the brain regulating pain perception and signaling). A third possibility not considered by the researchers is that these therapies influence divine healing energy.

Fifteen clinical studies were included that performed biofield therapies both during and after conventional cancer treatment. The review concluded that most of the evidence from the studies support reducing cancer-related pain, depression, and persistent fatigue through biofield therapies. Moreover, the review pointed out that preclinical cancer models suggest that biofield therapies may even have an effect on clinical biomarkers of cancer tumors. Suppression of DNA synthesis and mineralization (signs of stopping cancer cell growth and division) in osteosarcoma, inhibition of cancer cell cycles and the promotion of cancer cell death in prostate and colorectal cancer cells, and prevention of the migration of breast cancer cells were all noted. Since there is no physiological explanation for these effects on cancer tumors, it is conceivable that the therapies activated divine energy healing networks.

As far as other health conditions are concerned, a few clinical studies have demonstrated promising results for cardiovascular disease CVD, based on increased HRV and reducing stress and anxiety, which are known to negatively impact CVD. Similar benefits, including improvements in heart rate homeostasis, were observed in rats. Positive results of biofield therapies were also mentioned for dementia and osteoarthritis. Overall, the narrow scope of research burdened by limitations in population size and methodology points to promising results using biofield therapies for a variety of health conditions and further suggests that divine energy is relevant regardless of the health condition being treated.

Witnessing Energy Transfer from Practitioners

Intriguingly, research does insinuate that energy transfer from practitioners to clients is measurable and observable. A study found that there was a significant 11 percent reduction in biophoton emission from the practitioner's hands after an energy healing session.[77] This represents a quantifiable change in the energy output of the practitioner. Additionally, a unique biophoton emission pattern was observed during each energy healing session. Lastly, some, but not all, clients emitted more biophotons from specific bodily regions, some in alignment with their intent, after an energy healing session. In the context of energy healing, the reduction in emitted biophotons could suggest that the practitioner's energy is being utilized or transformed during the session. The reduction in biophoton emission may also point to an underlying mechanism through which energy healing might operate. For instance, it could indicate that the practitioner's body is engaging in processes like calming or grounding itself while transferring healing energy to the patient. These findings might reveal important information about the therapeutic partnership in terms of quantum (or quantum-like) entanglement—where two or more particles become deeply connected, regardless of the distance between them.

The Quantum Tapestry: Exploring Cellular Memory, Consciousness, and the Divine Connection

There is some evidence indicating quantum entanglement between tissues and blood components removed from subjects, as well as the influence of psychological states, emotions, and experiences on physiological processes. It seems that cells, blood, and tissues can retain "memory" of emotional states or traumatic experiences, which can impact health. For example, personality changes, memory transfer, and even lifestyle changes have been observed following organ transplants.[78] One study showed that 38 percent of heart transplant recipients exhibited characteristics partially similar to those of their donors.[79] Changes in food preferences that aligned more closely with their donor were commonly reported. Other recipients reported dreams that were not their own, hearing voices, and being more thoughtful or civilized. These findings suggest a profound connection between consciousness, cellular memory, and quantum phenomena, pointing to the possibility that divine energy weaves through all living systems, uniting physical and spiritual realms in the process of healing and transformation.

Some theories suggest a concept of "body memory" where physical tissues might hold traces of past experiences despite being separated from the body. This concept may not be as weird as you think because neuronal networks stored in the hippocampus facilitate both memory recall and hypothetically, these memories could be transferred to cells outside the nervous system. Think of "body memory" as a smartphone syncing its data to the cloud. When you take a photo on your phone, it's stored in both your device and the cloud, allowing you to access it anytime, even if you lose the phone. Similarly, the brain (like the phone) may record memories in the hippocampus, while the physical tissues (like the cloud) could retain traces of those experiences even when separated from the body, allowing for a kind of memory presence beyond the central nervous system. After all, our sense of self and identity is fundamentally based on knowledge obtained from several psychophysiological senses accumulated in cells, which are stored as implicit memory to uphold that sense of self in perpetuity.

When a memory is recalled, the hippocampus (and other parts of the brain involved in memory) can release neurotransmitters, which are chemical messengers that transmit signals between neurons. Some of these neurotransmitters can also affect cells outside the nervous system. For example, neurotransmitters can enter the bloodstream and influence various physiological processes, potentially impacting cellular behavior in peripheral tissues. Moreover, the brain communicates with the body through hormones. Stressful or emotionally charged memories can lead to the release of hormones such as cortisol and adrenaline from the adrenal glands. These hormones travel through the bloodstream and can affect countless processes in different tissues, influencing cellular responses throughout the body. It is possible that memories based on interaction with these neurotransmitters and hormones remain in peripheral cells long-term.

Continuing with the smartphone analogy, when you recall a memory—like opening a photo on your cloud—you trigger specific processes that bring that image to the forefront. In the brain, this involves the release of neurotransmitters, akin to downloading data to your device. These neurotransmitters act as chemical messengers that not only enhance communication between neurons but can also tap into the wider network of your body.

Just as a photo you open might remind you to send a message to a friend, those neurotransmitters can spill into the bloodstream and influence various physiological processes, impacting how different cells in your body behave. Likewise, recalling particularly intense or stressful memories can be like sending an emergency alert to your device; the brain releases hormones like cortisol and adrenaline, which then circulate through your body, affecting numerous functions in various tissues.

Over time, just as certain memories might linger on your device even after you've put it down, it's possible that the effects of these neurotransmitters and hormones leave lasting imprints in peripheral cells. These imprints could reflect the emotional weight of past experiences, subtly shaping the physical response of your body long after the moment has passed.

There is an emerging interest in how memories might influence gene expression through microRNAs and epigenetic mechanisms. Some studies suggest that the experience of learning and memory can lead to changes in gene expression patterns that may be reflected in cells throughout the body. MicroRNAs, which are small non-coding RNA molecules, can be released from neurons into circulation and potentially influence the behavior of distant cells. This can lead to epigenetic changes that influence how cells respond to their environment, effectively encoding some aspects of the memory experience at the cellular level.

Back to comparing cellular and body memories to a smartphone, think of your memories as not just files on a device but as software updates that enhance the phone's performance and features. When you download a significant update, it doesn't just change one app; it can affect how the entire system operates.

In this context, the experience of learning and memory can be likened to those updates influencing the underlying code of the phone's operating system. MicroRNAs are like small patches of code that are sent out from the main application (the brain) into the wider network (the body) whenever you access or engage with those memories. They travel through the system (in this case, your bloodstream) and communicate with other applications (cells throughout your body), adjusting how they function based on past experiences.

These microRNAs can lead to changes in how certain genes are expressed, much like how a software update can alter the settings or features of individual apps. This gene expression and the resulting epigenetic changes allow cells to adapt their responses to their environment, effectively encoding aspects of your memory at a cellular level, just as updates can track user preferences and habits to personalize functionality.

In essence, every time you learn something or recall a memory, you're not just accessing files; you're rewriting part of the system, allowing your body to respond in ways that reflect both past experiences and the adaptations they necessitated, creating a lasting impact that shapes how you function moving forward.

Memory can also manifest through interactions between the nervous system and immune cells. For instance, repeated learning or exposure to specific stimuli might lead to long-term changes in immune cell populations, which could be considered a form of memory stored within the immune system. Stressful memories, for example, can lead to changes in immune cell function, which may reflect a form of memory encoding outside of the nervous system. While direct transfer of memory recall from the hippocampus to cells outside the nervous system is an oversimplification of complex physiological processes, there are various pathways through which memories can influence tissue behavior and cellular responses throughout the body.

This cellular memory or deep connection with divine energy that unifies living things was also witnessed in experiments performed by Dr. Robert O. Becker in the 1970s. His both famous and infamous experiments demonstrated that tissue or blood removed from a subject can still respond to the experiences of the person from whom the blood or tissue was taken. He identified these changes by using live blood analysis (LBA). LBA, also known as live cell analysis or dark-field microscopy, is a controversial technique in which a drop of blood is observed under a specialized microscope in real time to assess the health of an individual. Unlike conventional blood tests, which often involve staining and analyzing dried samples in a lab, LBA examines fresh, unstained blood immediately after it's drawn. This allows for the visualization of living components such as red and white blood cells, platelets, plasma, and other structures in their natural state. Live blood analysis is commonly used by alternative and complementary medicine practitioners to provide insights into nutritional status, oxidative stress, immune function, digestive health, circulatory health, and the vitality of the blood, which reflects the body's overall energetic health.

Dr. Becker, an orthopedic surgeon and pioneer in bioelectric medicine, observed changes in the behavior of white blood cells when a person was exposed to stressful stimuli, even after the blood sample had been physically separated from their body. In this experiment, white blood cells displayed altered responses, such as increased activity, as if "sensing" the emotional state of their donor despite being removed from the body's direct influence. This suggested a form of communication or connection between the individual and their cells that defied conventional scientific explanations at the time.

Other researchers have explored similar phenomena, among others in studies in quantum biology and the biofield sciences. For instance, experiments conducted by Dr. Cleve Backster in the 1960s on plant and human cells revealed comparable results.[80] Backster's research involved attaching a polygraph to a plant leaf, whereupon he claimed to observe changes in the plant's electrical resistance when it was subjected to potential harm or stress. In humans, Backster demonstrated that cells removed from the human body, such as leukocytes (white blood cells), exhibited measurable electrical changes when the donor experienced emotional stimuli, such as stress or fear, even when separated by significant distances. These findings suggest a potential quantum or energetic entanglement that remains unexplained by classical biology but lends credence to the existence of divine energy unifying all living things.

While still a topic of debate in mainstream science, these experiments hint at the presence of a unified, interconnected system in which consciousness, emotional states, and biological processes are intricately linked. These observations could deepen our understanding of how divine energy or subtle energetic fields contribute to health, healing, and the profound connection between mind and body.

Stimulating Qi Through Acupuncture and Acupressure

Of the above-mentioned therapies, the benefits of acupuncture and acupressure have perhaps been most researched. Both of these modalities are rooted in the concept of balancing the body's energy flow, often referred to as Qi (pronounced *chi* in English) or life force, which matches closely with the idea of harnessing divine energy for healing. These practices aim to stimulate specific points on the body, known as acupoints, to regulate energy pathways, or meridians, and restore harmony within the body's systems.

Acupuncture and acupressure may influence biophoton emission by promoting cellular communication and coherence.

Research suggests that stimulating acupoints can enhance light communication within the body, reflecting an alignment with divine energy that supports natural healing processes.[81] Studies show that acupuncture can improve HRV,[82] an indicator of autonomic nervous system balance. By reducing stress and promoting relaxation, these therapies harmonize the heart and mind, facilitating a state of physiological coherence often associated with divine energy. Acupuncture and acupressure may help realign disrupted vibrational frequencies in the human body by clearing energy blockages and enhancing the flow of Qi, resonating with the concept of divine energy as a harmonizing force. Lastly, both acupressure and acupuncture interact directly with the human biofield. Acupoint stimulation is thought to refine the biofield's energy patterns, enabling the body to better absorb and integrate divine energy for physical, emotional, and spiritual healing. By influencing these interconnected aspects of energy and physiology, acupuncture and acupressure serve as powerful tools for channeling divine energy, promoting balance, and supporting the body's innate healing capabilities.

The preponderance of evidence in both humans and animals points to acupoints possessing characteristics of low electrical resistance and high electrical conductance.[83] Lower electrical resistance at acupoints may indicate a smoother flow of energy through the body's meridians. This balanced energy flow is believed to promote overall health and well-being. High electrical conductance at acupoints may enhance their responsiveness to various forms of stimulation—whether that's through acupuncture needles, pressure, heat, or electrical pulses. This heightened responsiveness helps activate the body's natural healing processes. By revealing how these points function and why they can be effective for promoting healing, we gain insights into how to harness their potential in both complementary and mainstream health practices.

The concept of a long-distance interstitial fluid (ISF) circulatory pathway originating from the acupoints in the extremities offers a fascinating connection between physical health and the flow of divine energy. This pathway aligns with the principles of traditional acupuncture and acupressure, which view acupoints as nodes of concentrated energy that influence the body's energetic and physical systems.

In health, ISF pathways are vital for nutrient delivery, waste removal, and communication between cells. When this circulation flows optimally, it supports homeostasis and cellular coherence, which are essential for healing and vitality. Research demonstrates that most acupoints in the extremities connect with one or more ISF flow pathways, forming a complex network, consisting of biological fluid (interstitial fluid composed of water, electrolytes, nutrients, waste products, and signaling molecules) and bioenergy.[84, 85] This intricate network designed like highways for fluid and energy, highlights how acupoints serve as vital gateways, harmonizing physical and energetic systems to support the body's natural healing processes and alignment with divine energy.

From the perspective of divine energy, these acupoints could serve as portals or conduits for this higher, harmonizing energy to enter and circulate throughout the body. By activating these points, whether through acupuncture, acupressure, or other modalities, one might amplify the flow of divine energy, aligning the body's physical and energetic systems. This can enhance the communication within the human biofield, potentially affecting measurable factors like HRV and vibrational frequency, which are markers of physiological and spiritual coherence. Thus, the ISF circulatory pathway might bridge physical processes with the metaphysical flow of divine energy, promoting genuine healing and balance.

Studies have shown that stimulating acupoints can trigger neural and hormonal responses, leading to various physiological effects.[86] Measurable endpoints could then prove that acupoint stimulation can reduce pain (endorphin and neurotransmitter release), combat stress (reduce cortisol), enhance immune function (cytokine regulation), and promote hormonal balance (sex hormones and others). A case study of people undergoing acupuncture treatment found that individuals "tended to have an increase in their HRV during treatment, after needling, and, in some instances, an increase in HRV over weeks to months."[87] This phenomenon points to the possibility that acupuncture treatments can help harmonize and regulate the flow of divine energy within an individual, creating a state of coherence that may endure well beyond the initial session. Consequently, acupuncture can be viewed not only as a therapeutic intervention but also as a practice that cultivates long-term well-being by nurturing the body's inherent capacity for balance and healing.

Reiki: Channeling Healing and Relaxing Energy

Reiki is a form of alternative therapy that originated in Japan in the early 20th century. It is based on the idea that there is a universal life force energy that flows through all living things, and this energy can be harnessed for healing. Practitioners of Reiki use their hands to channel this energy into the recipient, promoting relaxation and healing. The name "Reiki" itself is derived from two Japanese words: "Rei" meaning "universal" and "Ki" meaning "life energy."

Reiki practitioners believe that they can channel divine energy to facilitate healing. This energy is deemed to have a higher vibrational frequency and can help harmonize and balance the recipient's energy fields. Reiki aims to raise the recipient's vibrational frequency, supporting emotional healing and physical wellness. Both the intent of the practitioner and the recipient's openness are considered crucial for the effectiveness of the treatment.

Some researchers suggest that Reiki may influence biophoton emissions, leading to enhanced cellular communication and physiological balance. Reiki practitioners believe that the biofield can become imbalanced due to physical or emotional stressors, and Reiki is used to restore balance and harmony in the biofield, promoting healing on multiple levels. The effects of Reiki on biofields have been investigated in an animal cell-based model. Mice intervertebral disc cells were treated with a ten-minute session of Reiki or sham Reiki on successive days. During treatment, the cells were placed in a box with a photon multiplier tube, which are extremely sensitive detectors of light in the ultraviolet, visible, and near-infrared ranges of the electromagnetic spectrum. Observation via the photon multiplier tube allowed the researchers to detect increased biophoton emission of the cells after Reiki, which exceeded the emission produced by sham treatment.[88] Since these cells are not susceptible to a placebo effect, this is remarkable evidence of a change in divine energy following Reiki therapy.

A review of thirteen peer-reviewed clinical studies found that eight of those studies demonstrated that Reiki was more effective than a placebo in activating the body's intrinsic healing potential to restore both mental and physical well-being.[89] Within this review, some of the studies showed that Reiki shifts autonomic nervous system function toward a state of coherence based on increased heart rate variability and body temperature without increases in cortisol. Reiki seems to move humans in the direction of relaxation, which is strongly associated with health and healing..[90] Again, this points to more evidence that Reiki balances the human biofield, strengthening the body's ability to heal itself through aligning with divine energy.

One clinical study sought to measure the effect of a single Reiki session on physical and psychological health..[91] The well-validated 20-item Positive and Negative Affect Schedule was used to assess a wide range of physical and psychological outcomes immediately prior to and after the Reiki sessions. A total of 1,411 Reiki sessions were performed by ninety-nine Reiki practitioners. Statistically significant improvements in pain, drowsiness, tiredness, nausea, appetite, shortness of breath, anxiety, depression, and overall well-being were observed.

A meta-analysis of randomized controlled clinical trials that included four studies with a total of 212 participants assessed the effects of Reiki on pain..[92] Included in the meta-analysis were trials evaluating pain associated with cancer, neuropathy, enlarged lymph nodes, ascites (abnormal build-up of fluid in the abdomen), labor and delivery, and cesarean section. Comparing Reiki groups with control groups demonstrated a small, non-statistically significant reduction in pain. The researchers concluded that Reiki was an effective complementary practice for pain relief. An additional review article that included seven studies evaluating Reiki's effects on pain and anxiety related to cancer, surgery, and aging determined that Reiki may be effective for both pain and anxiety..[93] Currently, larger studies with better methodologies are necessary to confirm the efficacy of Reiki for pain, but the findings are trending toward positive effects.

Interest in using Reiki for mental and emotional conditions is also growing. A Cochrane Database review of three studies using Reiki for pain or depression concluded there is "insufficient evidence to say whether or not Reiki is useful for people over 16 years of age with anxiety or depression or both."[94] However, since the review was published, a new study found Reiki effective in reducing preoperative anxiety and in preventing it from increasing.[95] These findings suggest that while more robust evidence is needed, Reiki holds promise as a complementary approach for alleviating anxiety and supporting emotional well-being, particularly in stressful situations like surgery.

Acute Coronary Syndrome (ACS) is a term used to describe a range of conditions—such as unstable angina or heart attack—that suddenly reduce blood flow to the heart muscle. This can lead to heart damage or a heart attack (myocardial infarction). Autonomic nervous system dysfunction, as measured by HRV, is a strong predictor of patient outcome after ACS. Indeed, medications like beta-adrenergic blockers are used to enhance parasympathetic nervous system tone and improve results after ACS. A clinical study evaluated whether Reiki could improve HRV in people recovering from ACS.[96] Participants in the study were randomized to receive Reiki, classical musical intervention, or basic rest (control group) while undergoing continuous ECG monitoring. Baseline high-frequency HRV was significantly improved when compared to music therapy or resting. Reiki treatment was also associated with increases in positive mood and reductions in negative states (stressed, angry, sad, frustrated, worried, scared, anxious). These findings suggest that Reiki may be improving healing and patient outcomes by channeling divine energy.

Reiki offers a profound connection to the universal life force energy that flows through all living beings, providing a pathway to harmonize the body, mind, and spirit. The evidence of increased biophoton emissions and shifts in autonomic nervous system function underscores the tangible effects of this ancient healing practice. By aligning the biofield with divine energy,

Reiki facilitates a state of relaxation and coherence, amplifying the body's natural healing potential.

Unlocking Vital Energy: Exploring the Transformative Power of Qigong for Holistic Healing

Qigong is a holistic practice from Chinese medicine that integrates physical postures, breathing techniques, meditation, and mental focus to cultivate and balance "qi" (or "chi"), which is the vital life energy believed to flow through the body. Qigong combines elements of philosophy, health, and spirituality, promoting physical, emotional, and spiritual well-being.

The key components of qigong include energy, physical movement, breathing, meditation, and mental focus. In qigong, qi is the fundamental life force or energy that sustains all living beings. Qigong aims to cultivate, balance, and harness this energy for health and vitality. It involves various gentle physical movements and postures that are designed to enhance flexibility, strength, and circulation. Breath is an essential aspect of qigong that helps to enhance the flow of qi. Practitioners often incorporate deep, rhythmic breathing to calm the mind and energize the body. Qigong includes meditation practices to cultivate mindfulness, increase awareness, and promote relaxation. Mental focus is used to direct the flow of qi and enhance the effectiveness of the practice.

Qigong can be broadly categorized into two main types: internal qigong and external qigong. Internal qigong emphasizes internal cultivation and the development of awareness, intention, and energy flow within the body. Generally, it involves meditation, breathwork, and visualization techniques designed to harmonize the mind, body, and spirit. In contrast, external qigong, like Tai Chi, concentrates on physical exercises performed for wellness, healing, or martial arts applications. It involves dynamic movements, forms, and exercises that build strength, flexibility, and coordination while promoting the flow of qi throughout the body.

Qigong is a versatile practice that encompasses a range of techniques for cultivating and balancing life energy. Whether focusing internally or externally, Qigong offers practitioners a holistic approach to health and well-being. It can be adapted to suit individual needs, making it accessible to people of all ages and fitness levels. As with any practice, consistency is key to experiencing its full benefits.

Magnetic fields are typically measured using devices called magnetometers or gaussmeters using a unit of measurement called a Gauss (mGauss). For example, the Earth's magnetic field is approximately 0.5 Gauss, a refrigerator magnetic 10–100 Gauss, and an MRI machine around 10,000–30,000 Gauss. The human body generates a very weak magnetic field in the range of 0.0000001 to 0.000001 Gauss. This biomagnetic field is the result of small electrical currents generated by neurons and muscle cells when they fire. While individual cells may generate small magnetic fields, their contributions do not add up to create a strong overall field in the human body. In 1992, researchers published a report in which they mentioned that they detected a biomagnetic field from the hand of a person practicing external qigong in the order of 0.001 Gauss.[97] The researchers concluded that a biomagnetic field this strong cannot be produced from internal body current alone. Furthermore, they posited that it may have originated from qi energy. Or, in other words, it was a remarkable display of divine energy.

Similarly, researchers discerned an extremely strong biomagnetic field from the head of two individuals practicing qigong breathing exercises.[98] One participant emitted a biomagnetic field at the level of 2–3 Gauss and the other 1.3 Gauss—significantly higher than the normal magnitude of the human biofield. Given that the orientation and geometric arrangement of tissues in the body diffuse and diminish the strength of biomagnetic fields, a pulse of this magnitude is incredible. They concluded that practicing qigong seems to stimulate an unusually large biomagnetic field emission.

Extraordinarily, enhancement of biophoton emission through non-contact healing has been observed in cucumbers..[99] Japanese researchers measured the intensity of biophotons using a super-sensitive camera that had an image intensifier. Three groups were included: a control cucumber slice, a cucumber slice exposed to heat (40 degrees C; 104 degrees F), and treatment cucumber slices consisting of three slices treated with laying on of hands (qigong for 15 to 30 minutes) and one by praying (a 5-minute prayer approximately four feet from the cucumber). No changes were observed in the control or thermally exposed cucumbers, but the healing groups experienced significant increases in biophoton emission. These findings help rule out that the increased biophotons observed were due to the transfer of heat from hands during the qigong therapy as the heated cucumber did not experience the same increases in emission. Results from this study highlight the profound influence of intentionality and divine energy on living systems, offering a glimpse into the unseen connections that unite consciousness, biology, and the healing power of light.

The effects of both internal and external qigong have also been measured through EEG. Comparison of EEG readings of qigong masters who were resting with their eyes closed and while practicing qigong showed clearly distinct brain activity during qigong..[100] Alpha activity changes predominantly in the anterior half of the brain were detected and alpha activity changes occurred silently in the posterior half of the brain. This suggests that qigong induces a unique brain state, not commonly experienced by individuals who don't practice the technique, associated with a state of deep relaxation and altered consciousness, which may lead to various physiological and psychological benefits. Other research showed similar shifts in brainwave activity consistent with this distinct brainwave pattern.[101, 102] Another study evaluated the differences between concentrative and non-concentrative qigong states via EEG and topographic mapping study.[103] Results from the study correlated a concentrative qigong state to frontal mid-line theta rhythm—a state seen during mental concentration. These findings suggest that qigong practices can induce a unique state of consciousness characterized by specific brainwave patterns, potentially contributing to its various physical and mental health benefits.

The exploration of magnetic fields and their interaction with the human body through practices like qigong reveals fascinating insights into the profound connection between energy, consciousness, and healing. The robust biomagnetic fields observed during qigong practice and the enhancement of biophoton emissions in living organisms suggest the influence of intentionality and divine energy at work. These findings not only challenge conventional understanding of biological processes but also underscore the revolutionary potential of aligning with higher energetic frequencies. By fostering states of deep relaxation, altered consciousness, and heightened vibrational energy, qigong serves as a bridge between the physical and spiritual realms, offering a pathway to healing that transcends traditional methods and invites us to explore the boundless possibilities of divine design.

Tapping into Divine Energy: The Power of Touch

Therapeutic touch, massage therapy, and healing touch are distinct practices that share some common principles, particularly in their focus on healing and well-being through physical touch. However, they differ in their techniques, philosophies, and intended outcomes.

Massage therapy involves the manipulation of soft tissues in the body, including muscles, fascia, tendons, and ligaments, using various techniques such as stroking, kneading, and pressing. There are various styles, including Swedish, deep tissue, sports, and trigger point therapy, each with its own techniques and benefits. Unlike therapeutic touch, which centers on energy work, massage therapy primarily targets physical structures to relieve tension, promote relaxation, improve circulation, and enhance overall physical health. However, there is still an underlying belief that energy can be exchanged between the therapist and the recipient during massage therapy. Massage therapists undergo specific training and are often required to have licensure or certification to practice professionally.

Therapeutic touch is a form of energy healing that involves the practitioner's hands being placed near or on the patient's body to promote healing and relaxation. Developed by Dolores Krieger in the 1970s, it is based on the belief that practitioners can channel healing energy toward the recipient. Practitioners seek to influence the patient's energy field or "biomagnetic field" to facilitate healing. Practitioners typically undergo specific training to develop sensitivity to energy fields and learn techniques to balance and clear them. It is often used to reduce stress, alleviate pain, and promote emotional well-being.

Healing touch is another energy-based practice similar in philosophy to therapeutic touch developed by Janet Mentgen, RN in the 1980s. It involves light or near-body touch to balance the energy field and promote healing. Healing touch is typically practiced within the context of nursing and holistic care. Healing touch practitioners focus on a holistic view of health, addressing physical, emotional, mental, and spiritual aspects of well-being.

Like therapeutic touch, healing touch practitioners claim to manipulate the human energy field using specific techniques intended to restore balance and promote healing. Practitioners receive specialized training in healing touch techniques and often seek additional certification.

All three practices aim to promote healing and well-being, reduce stress, and improve overall quality of life. Each involves some form of touch or near-touch as a mechanism for facilitating healing. Healing Touch and Therapeutic Touch place a greater emphasis on energy healing and fields, whereas massage therapy is more grounded in anatomy and physiology, focusing more heavily on the physical bodies and structures rather than energy fields. Each practice can be effective for various needs and preferences, and many people benefit from incorporating elements of each into their wellness routines.

While there's been growing interest in the potential benefits of massage and its connection to the human biofield, scientific research specifically linking massage to the human biofield is limited, maybe because of its lower emphasis on energy healing. Nevertheless, the concept of transference suggests an energy exchange can occur between the therapist and the recipient during massage. Transference, in the context of massage therapy, refers to the phenomenon where emotions, feelings, and energy are exchanged or influenced between the therapist and the client during a massage session. This concept is rooted in psychology, particularly in the therapeutic relationship established between a client and a therapist, and it can manifest in several ways during massage therapy.

Emotional transference occurs when a client transfers feelings, memories, or unconscious desires onto the massage therapist. This could stem from past experiences, relationships, or expectations about care and touch. A client may feel deep trust, dependency, or even resistance toward the therapist, which can reflect their past relationships or unresolved emotions. Conversely, clients may project positive feelings such as gratitude or admiration. A therapist can also transfer positive or negative energies and emotions, making it important for the therapist to be in a healthy mental and emotional state while performing massage.

The exchange of unseen energy between the therapist and the client can influence the emotional and physical outcomes of the session. Practitioners believe that physical touch can transmit energy, leading to sensations of relaxation, tension release, or even emotional expression. Clients may experience this as a feeling of warmth, calm, or heightened awareness. Conversely, negative energy can also be transferred, resulting in discomfort or unease. Transference plays a significant role in shaping the therapeutic experience and contributes to the emotional dynamics at play during a session. By understanding, recognizing, and managing transference, both clients and therapists can enhance the effectiveness of the therapy, promote healing, and foster a supportive and transformative experience.

Because it is rooted more in energy healing, healing touch has more empirical evidence than massage in relation to directing divine energy for healing. A 2020 study found that healing touch reduced both pain and agitation in adults admitted to intensive care units.[104] The researchers noted improvements in objective hemodynamic measures (blood pressure, heart rate, cardiac output, and vascular resistance), resulting in a calmer state. While the primary endpoints confirm positive changes in vital signs after healing touch, the findings are also suggestive that energy healing practices can have measurable physiological effects.

Another study compared the benefits of healing touch to oncology massage for cancer pain relief.[105] Both healing touch and oncology massage provided immediate pain relief, with oncology massage being slightly more likely to provide pain improvement except in people reporting severe pretherapy pain. Other researchers demonstrated that healing touch improved overall vitality and physical function and reduced pain in seventy-eight women undergoing radiation therapy for gynecological cancers.[106] These conclusions suggest that energy-based therapies like healing touch can offer significant benefits for cancer patients, including pain relief and improved quality of life, complementing traditional medical treatments.

Post-traumatic stress disorder (PTSD) remains a significant challenge in returning military personnel, first responders, survivors of assault or abuse, and people who experienced disturbing accidents or disasters. A randomized controlled clinical trial demonstrated that healing touch with guided imagery was more effective than standard treatment in relieving PTSD among combat-exposed active duty military.[107] Therapists employed three distinct techniques of healing touch: Chakra Connection, which involves methods along the body designed to encourage the flow of vital energy; Mind Clearing, which consists of techniques applied to the head aimed at fostering mental relaxation; and Chakra Spread, an advanced method typically used for clients with more severe symptoms, focused on facilitating profound healing for emotional and physical distress. Not only were PTSD symptoms improved, but depression and cynicism diminished, and mental quality of life was enhanced. A different clinical trial reported that healing touch significantly reduced anxiety and length of stay at the hospital among people recovering from coronary bypass surgery.[108] Conclusions from these studies suggest that energy-based therapies like healing touch can be a valuable tool in addressing the complex challenges of PTSD and other trauma-related conditions, offering hope for those seeking relief and healing.

The empirical evidence supporting healing touch as an energy-based modality continues to reveal its profound potential in facilitating the flow of divine energy for healing. From reducing pain and agitation in intensive care patients to alleviating PTSD symptoms and enhancing vitality during cancer treatment, healing touch demonstrates how intentional energy work can bridge the gap between physical and spiritual restoration. Healing touch not only supports the body's innate healing processes but also fosters a deeper sense of peace and alignment. These findings affirm that healing touch is more than a therapeutic technique—it is a testament to the Creator's provision of tools to harmonize the body, mind, and spirit, empowering individuals to experience His life-changing power in their healing journey.

Therapeutic touch has a similar modest amount of research exploring its benefits. Its research started all the way back in the 1970s when brain activity was monitored via EEG while participating in therapeutic touch healing.[109] Therapeutic touch was compared to meditation and both practices induced a state of relaxation and altered consciousness, characterized by increased alpha and theta wave activity. Based on changes in beta brainwave activity, therapeutic touch seemed to alter consciousness in favor of alertness and focus. As explored in this study, the findings suggest that these practices can have a positive impact on mental and emotional well-being.

Another study concluded that therapeutic touch healers may have the ability to generate anomalous electrostatic phenomena—unusual or unexpected electrical charges or discharges that don't conform to well-understood physical laws—and these phenomena may be responsible for the healing effects of therapeutic touch.[110] The researchers measured the electrostatic potential of therapeutic touch healers using a sensitive electrometer. They found that the healers generated numerous body potential surges, with an average of two surges per minute. The surges were typically 44 volts DC (direct current) in amplitude. For comparison purposes, an AA battery produces about 1.5 volts DC and a car battery 12 volts DC. It is plausible that these scientists were witnessing and measuring the healing force of divine energy in real time during the experiment.

A 1993 study explored the potential psychoimmunologic effects of therapeutic touch on both practitioners and recently bereaved recipients.[111] Four to seven therapeutic touch sessions per subject were performed in a two-week period, which produced a greater mind-body connection and changes in the number of suppressor T cells when compared to their baselines. Similarly, a 2010 study noted changes in natural killer cell activity after therapeutic touch.[112] Additionally, decreased pain and cortisol levels were observed in the participants who received therapeutic touch while recovering from vascular surgery. Since the immune system plays a crucial role in both physical (e.g., inflammatory response, infection-fighting, and tissue repair) and psychological (e.g., neuroimmune connection, inflammation control, and stress response) healing processes, adaptations in its functions following energy healing can be interpreted as activating divine energy in the body.

A review article that included six clinical trials found that therapeutic touch generally improves health status in people with cancer.[113] Reduction in nausea, pain, stress, anxiety, and fatigue were discussed, as well as improvement in mood, mental health, and quality of life. Improvements in biological parameters were also seen, such as reduced blood pressure, heart rate, and respiratory rate. Therapeutic touch can be a valuable complementary therapy for cancer patients, offering potential benefits for physical, emotional, and psychological well-being, according to this research.

Therapeutic touch has also been evaluated as a complementary treatment for dementia. A randomized, double-blinded controlled trial compared the response to therapeutic touch among adults with responsive behaviors in dementia.[114] Responsive behaviors in dementia are actions, words, or gestures that a person with dementia uses to communicate a need or express discomfort. These behaviors can manifest as aggression, agitation, wandering, restlessness, hallucinations, paranoia, or withdrawal. They often arise due to unmet needs, such as pain, hunger, thirst, or boredom, or as a result of confusion or fear. Participants were divided into three groups: therapeutic touch, placebo (sham therapeutic touch), and control (standard care). The therapeutic touch group was the only group whose behavior improved during the treatment according to Revised Memory and Behavior Check scores. These findings remind us that therapeutic touch may be a promising complementary therapy for managing responsive behaviors in individuals with dementia, potentially improving their quality of life and reducing caregiver burden.

Back pain is a debilitating condition that frequently drives individuals to seek medical attention, severely impacting their overall quality of life. A pilot clinical study conducted for three months compared therapeutic touch to standard pharmacological pain management on back pain among adults in a neurological pain unit.[115] Participants in the therapeutic touch group received four therapeutic touch sessions on four consecutive days. Pain improvement of 45.6 percent (the Quebec Back Pain Disability Scale) and 43.0 percent (Numeric Pain Rating Scale) was achieved respectively in the therapeutic touch group. These are remarkable reductions in pain from a noninvasive technique that may represent reducing blockages of divine energy in the body to allow healing to occur.

A systemic review critically evaluated data from clinical trials involving the effectiveness of therapeutic touch as a comprehensive tool to reduce anxiety caused by various diseases.[116] A total of six articles were included and assessed in which it was demonstrated that therapeutic touch positively affects anxiety, pain, nausea, fatigue, and patients' quality of life. The researchers concluded that therapeutic touch "can improve health status of patients experiencing anxiety in various diseases such as cancer, heart diseases, stroke hypertension, anxiety, and depression."

Considering the growing body of research on therapeutic touch, it becomes increasingly evident that this practice may serve as a conduit for divine energy, facilitating healing in profound and measurable ways. From its impact on immune function and brainwave activity to its ability to alleviate pain, reduce anxiety, and enhance overall quality of life, therapeutic touch exemplifies the seamless interplay between body, mind, and spirit. These findings suggest that when we engage in practices like therapeutic touch, we may be tapping into the infinite power of divine energy to remove blockages and restore balance. As science continues to explore these ancient principles through modern methodologies, it underscores a timeless truth: the Creator has endowed His creation with tools for healing that transcend our understanding, inviting us to partner with Him in the sacred process of restoration and renewal.

Pranic Healing

Pranic Healing is a holistic healing technique that focuses on harnessing and manipulating the life force energy, or "prana," that exists in and around us. Developed by Master Choa Kok Sui in the late 20th century, pranic healing is based on the belief that our physical, emotional, and mental well-being is influenced by the flow and balance of energy within and around the body.

Prana is considered the vital energy that sustains life. It can be found in the air we breathe, sunlight, and even the food we consume. The balance and quality of this energy affect health and well-being. According to Pranic Healing, the human body has an energy body (also called the aura) that surrounds and interpenetrates the physical body. This energy body is composed of energy centers or chakras that correspond to different physical and emotional aspects of health. Illness, stress, and negative emotions are believed to cause blockages or imbalances in the energy body, which can manifest as physical ailments or emotional distress. Pranic healing aims to identify and remove these blockages to restore harmony. A pranic healing practitioner seeks to stimulate healing through two main steps: cleansing and energizing. Cleansing involves the removal of stagnant or negative energy from the patient's energy body using sweeping techniques, often performed with the hands without physical contact. After cleansing, the practitioner then directs fresh prana into the affected areas, replenishing and revitalizing the energy flow.

A qualitative meta-synthesis collected data from studies that looked at a range of effects on prana that occurred while receiving biofield therapies.[117] Subtle energy experiences that took place when practicing pranic energy perception and receiving any kind of biofield therapy included awareness of body temperature variation, a sensation of energy flow through the body, physical or tactile sensations of energy (tingling in the extremities, heaviness in the hand or body, electric sensations, sensations of vibration or floating), and a kind of attraction of magnetic sensation. The synthesizing of participants' experiences during pranic energy sessions supports the notion that a person can feel and experience subtle energy flow during sessions.

Other researchers instead focused on the pranic healing practitioners themselves, measuring HRV while performing meditation.[118] Both low and high-frequency components of HRV increased and total HRV was significantly higher. This suggests that guiding divine energy creates a dynamic interaction and balance between the sympathetic and parasympathetic nervous systems that can be measured via HRV.

While these studies offer intriguing glimpses into the potential effects of pranic healing, it's crucial to acknowledge that the field is still in its infancy. The evidence base remains limited, and further rigorous scientific research is necessary to substantiate these claims. As we delve deeper into the realm of subtle energy and consciousness, it's imperative to maintain a balanced perspective and open mind, recognizing that divine energy can be directed using many different techniques despite limited current evidence.

Johrei: Harnessing Divine Energy for Holistic Healing and Spiritual Purification

Johrei is a spiritual energy healing practice that originated in Japan during the early 20th century and was founded by the Japanese spiritual teacher Mokichi Okada, also known as Meishusama. The term "Johrei" translates to "purification of spirit," reflecting the practice's focus on healing not just physical ailments but also emotional and spiritual well-being through the transmission of divine energy.

It is practiced based on several key principles. Central to Johrei is the belief in a universal life force or divine energy that can be harnessed for healing. Practitioners believe this energy flows through the body and can be purified and directed for the healing of oneself and others. Johrei emphasizes purification of the spirit as a pathway to health. It posits that negative thoughts, emotions, and accumulated spiritual impurities can lead to physical and emotional distress. Healing involves cleansing these impurities to restore balance and harmony. Johrei practitioners use a hand-gesturing technique to channel divine energy toward a recipient. This is typically done in a seated or standing position, where the practitioner holds their hands in specific postures to facilitate the flow of energy. The recipient absorbs this energy, which is believed to help alleviate various physical, emotional, and spiritual issues.

Johrei is not only about healing but also aims for personal and collective spiritual growth. Practitioners are encouraged to adopt a lifestyle that includes meditation, ethical living, and service to others to deepen their connection to divine energy and enhance their healing capabilities. Lastly, Johrei places a strong emphasis on community. Practitioners gather in groups for collective healing sessions and community service, fostering a sense of interconnectedness and mutual support.

Japanese researchers sought to validate Johrei in the 1990s by conducting experiments that measured changes in consciousness by recording EEG, changes in autonomic nervous system function (pulse and blood pressure), changes in meridians, and changes in the discharge patterns of leaves under healing using Kirlian photography—a specific imaging technique that captures electrical coronal discharges..[119] Kirlian photography is a method used to display colorful, luminous patterns that are interpreted as a representation of the object's energy field or life force. It was found that Johrei practitioners triggered changes in the activity of meridians, synchronous changes in EEG for both the healer and recipient, and increases in corona discharges of leaves. While they declined to make a statement about the origin of healing energies, they did state the existence of subtle energies was clearly demonstrated.

A small study evaluated the effects of Johrei among people experiencing functional chest pain of noncardiac origin.[120] Participants in the intervention group received eighteen Johrei sessions from a practitioner during six weeks. There was a significant reduction in chest pain pre- and post-treatment in the Johrei group. The findings are suggestive of participant expectation having an impact on outcome and do show that Johrei may have a role in improving functional chest pain symptoms.

The evidence emerging from studies on Johrei healing highlights the intricate interplay of subtle energies in promoting physiological and emotional well-being. The synchronous changes in EEG activity between healer and recipient, the activation of meridians, and the striking corona discharges observed through Kirlian photography underscore the tangible effects of this spiritual healing practice. While researchers refrained from identifying the origin of these healing energies, the results strongly suggest that Johrei facilitates the flow of divine energy, offering comfort and relief to those in need.

Energy Kinesiology: Bridging Mind, Body, and Spirit for Holistic Healing

Energy kinesiology is a holistic health practice that combines insights from applied kinesiology and energy medicine. It is based on the understanding that physical, emotional, and spiritual well-being are interconnected and that imbalances in one area can affect the others. Practitioners use muscle testing as a diagnostic tool to pinpoint areas of imbalance or dysfunction within the body, allowing them to identify the root causes of health issues rather than merely addressing symptoms.

Muscle testing involves assessing the strength or weakness of specific muscles in response to various stimuli (e.g., thoughts, physical touch, or substances). This is used to determine the body's energetic responses and identify areas that may require attention. Similar to concepts in traditional Chinese medicine, energy kinesiology operates on the premise that there are pathways (meridians) through which life energy (qi) flows. Blockages or disruptions in these pathways can lead to physical and emotional problems. Energy kinesiology employs various techniques to restore balance, including physical exercises, acupressure, breath work, affirmations, and visualization. These methods aim to enhance the flow of energy and promote healing. By relating to the use of divine energy for healing, it emphasizes holistic approaches that consider the mind, body, and spirit. This practice not only seeks to restore health but also empowers individuals to connect with their own inner healing resources, which may be enhanced through the invocation of divine energies.

Energy kinesiology aims not only to restore optimum flow of energy throughout the body but also to enhance the body's biofield. This biofield is intimately connected to the human body and contains information or instructions vital to coordinating life-sustaining functions. Fascinatingly, Dr. Robert Becker observed that frogs, which can regenerate new limbs, exhibited a positive electrical potential across an amputated arm that gradually faded to zero as the stump healed.[121] Even stranger, the frogs grew a new limb when Becker artificially applied a negative potential to the site of the frog's amputated limb. Restoration of energy flow along body meridians may positively influence the human biofield. Research supporting the use of energy kinesiology is currently lacking, but positive experiences by countless individuals suggest that it is worthy of further exploration.

Reflexology: Tapping into Healing Energy Through the Body's Reflex Points

Reflexology is a holistic therapy that involves applying pressure to specific points on the feet, hands, and ears, which correspond to different organs, systems, and structures of the body. The premise is that these reflex points are linked to various areas within the body through nerves and energy channels, and stimulating them can help promote relaxation, balance, and healing. It is reported that the feet have about 200,000 nerve endings per foot, the ears thousands each, and the hands approximately 17,000 touch receptors and free nerve endings per square inch, dwarfing the nerve endings found in other areas of the body like the torso. Reflexology is based on the principles of energy flow and encourages the body's natural healing processes.

Many reflexologists believe that the practitioner's energy can influence the effectiveness of the therapy. By cultivating a state of presence, mindfulness, and intention, practitioners can create a space where divine energy can flow, facilitating healing for the client. Like other energy healing modalities, reflexology acknowledges that the body operates on various vibrational frequencies. Practitioners may align their work with higher frequencies—often associated with divine energy—to enhance the healing experience and support the client's energetic and spiritual alignment. Just as divine energy is thought to resonate at a higher frequency of love, compassion, and healing, reflexology utilizes similar concepts of resonance to connect with the patient. Through this practice, both practitioners and clients have the opportunity to engage with divine energy, facilitating a deeper level of healing and personal empowerment.

Researchers explored the effects of reflexology on HRV in twenty healthy subjects in two separate studies.[122, 123] The ECG of the participants was taken while in a relaxed sitting position for twenty minutes. Participants then received reflexology just below the toes via a mechanical reflexology device for another twenty minutes. The researchers measured HRV entropy. Entropy is a measure of how much disorder or randomness there is in a system. In the case of your heart rate, it measures how much your heart rate changes over time with higher HRV equating to greater variability and complexity. The more your heart rate changes (higher HRV), the more entropy there is in your heart rhythm. The researchers noted significant changes in HRV entropy after reflexology. High HRV often reflects a more complex and adaptable cardiovascular system, which aligns with the concept of entropy as a measure of disorder (in a positive sense, indicating a flexible and responsive system). Furthermore, the researchers concluded that reflexology stimulation can increase the complexity of the HRV signal to a healthier state.

More recently, Scottish researchers used reflexology to stimulate the heart reflex point on the foot of eleven healthy men and monitored any changes in cardiac function in response.[124] Trained therapists performed reflexology on the heart reflex for about 4.5 minutes, applying light to moderate pressure. An immediate modest change in cardiac output—the amount of blood pumped by the heart in one minute and a crucial indicator of the heart's efficiency in supplying oxygen and nutrients to body tissues—occurred during the left foot treatment. These findings suggest that reflexology to the upper half of the left foot may modestly improve cardiovascular parameters in healthy individuals.

While the potential connection between reflexology and divine energy presents a fascinating area of exploration, it remains a largely theoretical concept that requires further scientific validation. Although anecdotal reports and spiritual traditions suggest that reflexology may influence energy flow and promote a deeper sense of connection to the divine, robust clinical research is warranted to substantiate these claims. Continued research could illuminate the mechanisms by which reflexology might interact with divine healing energy, offering a clearer understanding of its role in holistic well-being. Until then, reflexology's impact on divine energy remains an intriguing possibility worthy of deeper inquiry.

The Healing Code®

The Healing Code book, written by Dr. Alex Loyd, is a self-help book that proposes a scientific and spiritual approach to healing. The book is based on the idea that emotional traumas and negative thoughts can create disruptions in the body's energy fields, leading to physical and psychological ailments. According to the book, the "Healing Code" is a specific sequence of thoughts, emotions, and prayers that can be used to restore balance to the body's energy fields—the crown, the forehead, the temples, and the back of the neck—promoting healing and relief from various ailments.

The book shares an energy model that consists of three main components:

- The Heart-Wall: a protective barrier created by emotional traumas that blocks the flow of love, light, and life force energy.
- The Negative Thoughts: thoughts and emotions that are stored in the Heart-Wall and create blockages in the body's energy fields.
- The Body's Energy Fields: the body's subtle energy fields that store memories, emotions, and experiences.

The book provides a step-by-step process for applying the "Healing Code" to release blockages and restore balance to the body's energy fields:

- Identify the negative thoughts and emotions associated with a specific issue or ailment.
- Use a specific sequence of thoughts, emotions, and prayers to "clear" the blockage in the Heart-Wall.
- Use visualization techniques to imagine the release of the blockage and the restoration of balance to the body's energy fields.
- Repeat the process daily for a specified period to achieve optimal results.

The book incorporates various principles and techniques from spirituality, meditation, and energy medicine, including:

- Forgiveness: releasing negative emotions and thoughts
- Gratitude: focusing on positive thoughts and emotions
- Visualization: using mental imagery to create desired outcomes
- Prayers: using spiritual language to connect with a higher power
- Energy centers: working with specific energy centers in the body

The book is mentioned here because it imparts another way to harness divine energy for healing. Many people have reported positive results from using "The Healing Code," while others have not had the same success. Nonetheless, the principles in the book are similar to those proposed in this work and involve eliminating emotional traumas that create blockages in the body's energy fields. Some people may find the book helpful in their personal healing journeys and use it as another tool to leverage divine energy for healing.

Crystal Healing: Employing Vibrational Energy for Holistic Transformation

Crystal healing is a holistic practice that involves using various crystals and gemstones to facilitate physical, emotional, and spiritual healing. The underlying belief is that each crystal has its own unique vibrational frequency and energy, which can interact with the human body's energy field to promote healing, balance, and well-being. Crystals are thought to resonate at specific frequencies due to their atomic structure. Each type of crystal has distinct properties and energies, which can affect the body and mind differently. For example, amethyst may be associated with tranquility and spiritual awareness, while rose quartz is often linked to love and emotional healing.

Crystals are frequently used to align and balance the body's energy centers that correspond to specific physical, emotional, and spiritual attributes. By placing specific crystals on or around these energy centers, practitioners aim to clear blockages and restore energy flow. Crystals may help align a person's energy field with the higher frequencies of love, light, and divine consciousness. The relationship between crystal healing and divine energy is evident in the way crystals are used to channel higher frequencies, align energy centers, and set intentions that resonate with spiritual principles.

Despite the upsurge in crystal healing popularity in recent years, scientific research has largely ignored this modality. In 2001, Christopher French and his team shared the findings of their research regarding crystal healing at the British Psychological Society Centenary Annual Conference in Glasgow. The investigation included eighty participants who held a real quartz crystal or fake quartz crystal while meditating. The researchers found that the effects and sensations reported by those who held real and fake crystals were no different. One finding of this study emphasizes the power of belief and the mind-body connection. Those who were primed beforehand to notice any sensations they felt while holding crystals were more likely to report a feeling of warmth in the hand and an increased feeling of overall well-being, regardless of whether they were holding a real or fake crystal. Furthermore, those who believed in the power of crystals were twice as likely as non-believers to report feelings from the crystals.

While crystal healing continues to captivate many as a tool for holistic well-being, its effectiveness remains largely anecdotal and rooted in personal belief systems. The findings from research, such as the study by Christopher French and his team, highlight the profound influence of belief and the mind-body connection in shaping individual experiences with crystals. This underscores the need for further scientific investigation to determine whether the effects of crystal healing extend beyond placebo responses. By deepening our understanding of how crystals interact with the body's energy field—or whether such interactions occur at all—future studies could either validate or refine this practice within the broader framework of complementary and alternative medicine. Until then, crystal healing remains an intriguing modality that thrives at the intersection of science, spirituality, and human perception.

Some may argue that the use of crystals is not in alignment with principles in Christianity, but the Bible would suggest otherwise. Moses and Aaron used physical objects—Moses' staff and Aaron's rod—to manifest God's will and power.[125] Moses invited the Israelites to look on a bronze serpent fastened to a pole for healing, which can be interpreted as teaching people about faith.[126] Elijah used his cloak to smite and divide waters so he and Elisha could cross on dry ground.[127] Similarly, others have used natural objects for access to revelation or as instruments to manifest God's work.[128, 129, 130] What this indicates is that objects created by God, and endowed with divine energy, can be harnessed by some of His children when necessary for His work.

As we conclude our exploration of energy healing techniques, it becomes clear that each modality, whether it be acupuncture, Reiki, or therapeutic touch, serves as a unique pathway to balance and harmonize the intricate web of energy that flows through our bodies. These practices, deeply rooted in ancient wisdom yet enhanced by modern understanding, reveal the profound interconnectedness between our physical, emotional, mental, and spiritual states. By harnessing the power of energy, each technique invites us to engage with our inner selves, facilitating true healing. As we navigate the complexities of life, these diverse approaches empower us to channel divine energy, promoting harmony, resilience, and personal transformation. Whether we seek relief from physical ailments or a serene mind, the journey through these energy-healing techniques offers us the tools to cultivate balance and fosters a greater connection to the universal energy that surrounds us. By embracing these modalities, we embark on a path of strength and vibrancy, ultimately guiding us toward a more harmonious and fulfilled existence.

Foot Zoning and Energy Healing

Foot zoning is a therapeutic practice based on the belief that the feet contain energy zones corresponding to various parts of the body. This practice operates on the premise that the feet act as a map or blueprint for the entire body, and by applying pressure or massaging specific zones, energy blockages can be cleared, allowing for a balanced flow of energy throughout the system.

Considered an advanced form of reflexology, and developed by Dr. Charles Ersdal of Norway, foot zoning views the body as an interconnected system rather than isolating it into distinct symptomatic areas. Like other energy healing techniques, it seeks to establish balance, improve the flow of divine energy, renew cells, and optimize body systems through the stimulation of signals on the feet. Each zone on the feet corresponds to a different area of the body—organs, glands, muscles, and even emotions. For example, a practitioner may work on the area of the foot linked to the liver to help detoxify the body or aid overall liver function. By stimulating specific foot zones, signals are sent to corresponding areas to restore healthy nervous system function, release emotional disturbances, balance hormones, and more.

The hands-on work of foot zoning is done gently, using light pressure or tapping to stimulate these energy zones. This practice promotes relaxation, reduces stress, and increases blood flow. Although the research specific to foot zone therapy is still emerging, its foundation in reflexology has opened avenues for understanding its potential health benefits. Additionally, many individuals report that foot zoning provides relief from various physical ailments and supports overall energy balance.

CHAPTER EIGHT

Connecting with Divine Energy Through Sound and Novel Technology

In the intricate tapestry of existence, sound emerges as one of the most profound elements, weaving its way into the very fabric of our healing journey. For centuries, various cultures have revered sound as a transformative force, capable of resonating with the vibrational frequencies that govern our physical, emotional, and spiritual well-being. Every living being—indeed, every atom—emanates its own unique melody, revealing a harmony that can either uplift or disrupt. As we explore sound therapy within the context of divine energy, we uncover not just a method of healing, but a powerful conduit to align ourselves with the universe's inherent wisdom. Through intentional sound practices, we engage in an ancient dialogue between our soul and the cosmos, embracing the potential to restore balance, transcend limitations, and unlock the divine energy that lies within us all.

In the quest for holistic healing, novel technologies have been introduced as revolutionary approaches to integrating the principles of energy medicine and human individuality. From bioresonance therapy, which facilitates a complex symphony of vibrations in cells, organs, and systems within the human body, to various light therapies that leverage non-ionizing radiation to facilitate healing on multiple levels, technology is exploring ways to heal by means of energy.

The Symphony of the Soul: Exploring Sound Therapy and Divine Energy

Sound has been recognized for centuries in various cultures and healing practices as a powerful tool for promoting healing and enhancing well-being. Everything in the universe, including our bodies, has a vibrational frequency. Sound is a type of vibration that can influence these frequencies, affecting our physical and emotional states. Certain sound frequencies are believed to resonate with different aspects of the body and spirit, promoting healing. For example, frequencies like 528 Hz are often associated with love and transformation. When a sound is produced, it can resonate with our body's energy centers, helping to clear blockages and harmonize energy flow. Different sounds can influence brain wave patterns. For instance, binaural beats—a technique that plays two slightly different frequencies in opposite ears—can promote relaxation, focus, or even meditative states. By harnessing the power of sound and its ability to align with our body's frequencies, we can unlock deeper healing and restore balance, promoting overall well-being on a physical, emotional, and spiritual level.

Based on this, a variety of sound healing practices have been utilized in both ancient and modern times. Music therapy uses music to improve mental and physical health. It can reduce stress, anxiety, and pain, promoting a sense of peace and happiness. Instruments like Tibetan singing bowls or gongs create soothing sounds that many believe help to ground the body, heal the mind, and connect with a higher state of consciousness. Even repeating specific sounds, words, or phrases can create a meditative state that connects individuals with a deeper sense of self and the universe, enhancing spiritual well-being. Engaging with calming sounds or uplifting music can trigger a relaxation response, create physiological and psychological coherence, and promote overall well-being. Sound unites the physical and metaphysical realms, acting as a catalyst for healing and transformation. By resonating with our bodies and emotions, sound helps us tap into divine energy, promoting homeostasis.

An observational study examined the effects of Tibetan singing bowl meditation on mood, anxiety, pain, and spiritual well-being.[131] Sixty-two men and women were asked to lie down in a half-circle or oblong-shaped configuration (depending on the space of the room) with their heads toward the musical instruments—Tibetan singing bowls, crystal singing bowls, gongs, cymbals, bells, didgeridoos, and other small bells. The Tibetan singing bowls were the major instruments used during the sessions, with the other instruments playing only five percent of each session. The participants were instructed by the lead musician to merely observe any sensations they felt without judging them and simply relax and enjoy the session. When compared with their pre-sound meditation state, participants reported significantly less tension, anger, fatigue, and depression. They also reported enhanced spiritual well-being. Interestingly, participants who had never experienced singing bowls experienced the greatest reduction in tension. This research suggests that high-intensity, low-frequency sounds and music can improve divine energy coherence.

Scientists hypothesize that the healing benefits of sound meditations may be due to alterations in brainwaves and HRV, binaural beats, and the sound vibrations interacting with the human biofield.[132, 133] During a sound meditation, brainwaves may significantly change from a normal or agitated state (such as beta waves) to an exceptionally relaxed brainwave state (such as theta or delta waves). When hearing a tone of one frequency in one ear and a different frequency in the other ear, your brain synchronizes (entrains) the tones to create an additional tone you hear. For example, if you play a 320 Hz tone in one ear and a 315 Hz tone in the other ear, the brain entrains to 5 Hz, which is the difference between the two tones. Entrainment captures the concept that if the brain can process and synchronize the auditory illusion created by two different frequencies into a coherent response, the body can similarly create a state of coherence that involves profound implications for healing. Physics states that there is no difference between energy and matter, and this can be applied to the human biofield. Sound vibrations may interact with this biofield to create an ideal environment for healing through divine energy.

Bioresonance Therapy: Restoring Harmony, Aligning Energy, and Unlocking the Body's Self-Healing Potential

Bioresonance therapy is a noninvasive, alternative treatment method that uses electromagnetic frequencies to detect and treat imbalances in the body. It emphasizes that each human being is unique; therefore, each condition a human experiences is unique to that person and must be treated distinctively. The therapy is based on the idea that every cell, organ, and system in the body emits specific electromagnetic frequencies. In a healthy state, these frequencies are harmonious, but illness or dysfunction can disrupt this harmony. By applying tailored electromagnetic signals, bioresonance aims to restore the body's natural balance, promoting healing and well-being.

Proponents of bioresonance therapy often view the electromagnetic frequencies it utilizes as a means to align the body with the universal or divine energy. This concept supports holistic perspectives that see the body as an interconnected system influenced by unseen forces such as light, energy, and vibration. By harmonizing cellular frequencies, bioresonance therapy could theoretically enable the body to better receive and utilize divine energy for healing.

Bioresonance therapy may influence biophoton emission. By restoring the natural electromagnetic balance in the body, bioresonance therapy may enhance the organization of these biophotons, improving cellular communication and energy flow. By reducing stress and promoting balance in the body's electromagnetic fields, bioresonance therapy may also increase HRV. The human biofield, or energy field, is believed to encompass and permeate the body, interacting with its physical, emotional, and spiritual aspects. Bioresonance therapy works directly on this field by correcting disruptions in its electromagnetic patterns. This harmonization of the biofield supports the body's natural healing mechanisms and may enhance the flow of divine energy. Lastly, bioresonance therapy is directly tied to vibrational frequency. Every organ and tissue has a unique vibrational signature, and bioresonance therapy aims to restore these frequencies to their optimal states. Bioresonance therapy offers a unique approach to healing by addressing the electromagnetic frequencies of the body. By doing so, it helps harmonize the body's overall vibrational frequency, promoting physical and emotional well-being.

To fully grasp this concept, think of the body as a complex communication network, like a city's electrical grid. Each cell, organ, and system is like a building, with wires (pathways) connecting them to ensure the smooth flow of power (energy) and information. In a well-functioning city, electricity flows efficiently, powering every building and enabling communication between systems.

When disruptions occur—like frayed wires, power surges, or outages—it can cause parts of the grid to malfunction, leading to confusion, inefficiency, or breakdowns. Bioresonance therapy works like an expert technician, diagnosing these disruptions and recalibrating the system. By restoring the proper flow of electricity and repairing the connections, it ensures the entire grid operates smoothly again, allowing the "city" (body) to function at its best.

A thought-provoking experiment was performed to assess whether bioresonance therapy impacted symptoms of various conditions of the nose, eye, respiratory system, skin, and gastrointestinal tract..[134] The study included 311 women and men aged from 2 to 76 years. After undergoing bioresonance therapy for twelve months, 90 percent of participants had no symptoms at all or showed significant improvement of their symptoms, regardless of the condition they were experiencing. Remarkably, 76.9 percent of participants experienced immediate relief of symptoms. These compelling results underscore the profound potential of bioresonance therapy to deliver rapid and lasting relief, offering a transformative approach to restoring health and harmony across a wide range of conditions.

Another study evaluated the effects of bioresonance therapy on major depression..[135] Three groups were formed from 140 participants: group one received solely bioresonance therapy, group two received pharmaceutical antidepressants with bioresonance therapy, and group three received solely antidepressants. What the researchers found was that bioresonance therapy accelerates the healing process and reduces major depressive disorder. Bioresonance therapy alone was more effective than antidepressants alone, with bioresonance therapy plus antidepressants showing the greatest improvement, suggesting a synergistic effect. Based on these results, it is possible that the bioresonance therapy enhanced electromagnetic frequencies in the body, potentially optimizing nerve signaling and reducing neuroinflammation to improve the response to the antidepressants. These two studies highlight the fact that bioresonance therapy can be effective for both physical and mental/emotional ailments. A highly possible explanation for this is that the therapy channels divine energy so the body can serve its purpose as a self-healer.

Harnessing Biophoton Technology: Innovative Tools for Focusing Divine Energy and Enhancing Self-Healing

Innovative technology is also being utilized to focus divine energy as a means of healing. Biofeedback devices focusing on measuring biophoton emissions aim to harness the principles of biophoton research to provide users with insights into their health and wellness. These devices are designed to collect data on the body's light emissions, which are associated with cellular processes and overall biological functioning. Researchers have linked changes in biophoton emissions to various health conditions, promoting the idea that monitoring these emissions could indicate shifts in biological processes related to health and disease.

Biofeedback devices often utilize highly sensitive photodetectors or photomultipliers to capture the weak light emissions from the body. These sensors can detect the very low intensities associated with biophotons, often in the range of a few photons per second. The detected biophoton emissions are then processed and analyzed through sophisticated algorithms. This analysis can identify patterns related to metabolic activity, stress levels, and overall vitality. Some advanced devices may utilize spectroscopic techniques to analyze the photon emissions more deeply, providing insights into the specific wavelengths emitted, which can be correlated with particular physiological states.

Many biofeedback devices provide real-time data on biophoton emissions. Users can observe their emission levels continuously or during specific activities, allowing them to identify changes in their energetic state. Feedback is typically provided through visual displays (graphs, color changes, etc.) or auditory signals. For instance, a user might see a change in light or hear tones that represent shifts in their biophoton emissions, indicating changes in their health status or energy levels. Users can often track their biophoton data over time, allowing them to recognize patterns or triggers related to their physical or emotional states. This historical data helps users make informed decisions regarding lifestyle changes or interventions and monitor their healing progress.

One example of this type of device is the Chiren 3.0, which is a sophisticated instrument developed by Johan Boswinkel for assessment and treatment with biophotons. It uses fiberoptic technology to conduct biophotons to and from the body and allows the immediate visualization of treatment effects. In a typical session, the practitioner assesses the body using a system similar to electroacupuncture to identify any disturbances in one or more organ systems. If a chaotic energy pattern is detected, the practitioner deploys a countersignal to a particular point, attempting to produce a coherent and healthy energy pattern. The individual receives biophotons through a glass rod held in one hand, which amplifies the coherent light and inverts (the opposite signal neutralizes the chaotic light) the damaging chaotic light. The resulting light is sent back to the body via a second glass rod held in the other hand. The same process of measurement and treatment is repeated on the feet. In short, the machine harnesses healthy coherent light produced by the body and directs it back into the body—millions of corrective cycles each second—to trigger the body's own self-healing ability.

Illuminating Healing: The Science of Light Therapy in Restoring Balance and Vitality

Light Therapy encompasses various therapeutic techniques that utilize specific wavelengths of light to promote healing, reduce pain, and enhance overall well-being. Among its various forms, Low-Level Laser Therapy (LLLT), Photobiomodulation (PBM), and Red-Light Therapy (RLT) are prominently studied methods. All three techniques involve the use of non-ionizing radiation to stimulate biological processes, potentially facilitating healing on multiple levels.

LLLT involves the application of low-intensity laser light to damaged tissues to promote healing, reduce inflammation, and alleviate pain. PBM is a related concept that refers to the use of light (including diode lasers and light-emitting diodes) to stimulate cellular processes. RLT is a specific form of light therapy that utilizes red and near-infrared light wavelengths (typically between 600 to 900 nanometers) to promote healing and overall wellness. Light therapies primarily function through the absorption of photons by chromophores, such as cytochrome c oxidase within mitochondria and calcium ion channels. This absorption triggers a cascade of cellular events, including increased ATP production, enhanced cellular metabolism, and reduced oxidative stress. Indeed, light therapy triggers a brief burst of reactive oxygen species, suggesting an increase in biophotons..[136] Subsequently, this process turns on many special proteins in the cells that help them stay alive, grow and multiply, move to where they're needed, and make new proteins. This therapeutic use of light aligns with the concept of divine energy, as it harnesses natural wavelengths to restore balance, vitality, and the body's innate ability to heal.

Some researchers believe that light therapy can interact with biological systems at the cellular level, influencing biophoton emissions. Evidence suggests that light therapy, particularly PBM, can promote the release of reactive oxygen species (ROS)—an indicator of increased biophoton emission—and other signaling molecules, thereby enhancing cellular communication and healing processes. Research indicates that light therapy can have positive effects on autonomic nervous system regulation, which can manifest as improved HRV. For example, studies have shown that PBM can reduce inflammation and promote relaxation, leading to increased HRV. The idea that light has a vibrational frequency relates to the concept that different wavelengths (colors) of light can influence biological systems in unique ways. Each wavelength has a specific energy associated with it, and this energy can interact with cellular processes. Certain frequencies of light can promote healing and energetic balance, paralleling notions of vibrational healing. It is also hypothesized that the interaction of light with the body could potentially enhance the flow of energy within the biofield, fostering physical and emotional healing.

PBM fosters coherence in divine energy according to preliminary research. It produces reactive oxygen species in healthy cells (amplifies divine energy to sustain health) but decreases reactive oxygen species in already stressed cells (prevents overwhelming the cell and allows divine energy to restore stability).[137] NF-κB (nuclear factor kappa-light-chain-enhancer of activated B cells) is a protein complex that plays a critical role in regulating the immune system, inflammation, and cell survival. Its importance for health lies in its ability to respond to various signals in the body and maintain balance in key processes, including tissue generation and repair, cancer prevention, chronic disease regulation, and inflammation control. More evidence of PBM fostering divine energy coherence is that the same research revealed that PBM activates NF-κB normal quiescent cells (resting cells in your body that are healthy and alive but are not actively growing, dividing, or doing a lot of work at the moment); on the other hand, it decreases the inflammatory factors associated with NF-κB in activated inflammatory cells. This dual regulation highlights how PBM harmonizes divine energy, promoting healing and balance by supporting healthy cellular function while calming overactive inflammatory responses.

Emerging research, particularly in photobiomodulation (PBM), supports the notion that specific wavelengths of light interact with the body in measurable ways, such as stimulating ATP production, reducing inflammation, and enhancing cellular communication. This scientific evidence parallels the idea of light as a conduit for divine energy, channeling specific frequencies to restore balance, promote healing, and connect individuals to a greater spiritual flow.

The Rejuvenating Effects of Red-Light Therapy on Healing and Cellular Energy

Red-light therapy (RLT) is a noninvasive treatment that utilizes specific wavelengths of light to promote healing and cellular function. It is based on the principle that light can penetrate the skin and influence biological processes at the cellular level, particularly in mitochondria, which are the energy-producing units of cells. RLT is often used to improve skin conditions, reduce inflammation, alleviate pain, and enhance overall tissue repair.

When red or near-infrared light is applied to the skin, it is absorbed by the mitochondria, leading to increased adenosine triphosphate (ATP) production, resulting in enhanced cellular energy and function. RLT helps reduce oxidative stress and inflammation, which can accelerate healing and tissue repair. It can also enhance circulation, delivering more oxygen and nutrients to tissues, further promoting healing.

Red-light therapy predominantly employs two specific ranges of wavelengths:

- Red light (600–700 nm): Commonly around 630 to 660 nm. This range is effective for superficial penetrations, making it ideal for skin conditions, wound healing, and promoting collagen production.
- Near-infrared light (700–900 nm): Commonly around 810 to 850 nm. This range penetrates deeper tissues and is effective for reducing pain and inflammation, promoting muscle recovery, and addressing joint issues.

Both red-light therapies operate under the premise that energy can flow and be manipulated in the body. Red-light therapy is viewed as a form of energy medicine, where light energy is harnessed to influence cellular behavior and promote healing. It leverages specific wavelengths that resonate with cellular structures, promoting optimal energy states within tissues.

Red-light therapy is a valuable tool in the realm of wellness and healing that can intersect with various energy healing modalities. By understanding the scientific foundations behind RLT and its wavelengths, practitioners can integrate it into holistic healing practices and complement other energy work aimed at balancing the body's energy fields and promoting overall health.

Similar to other forms of light therapy, RLT may influence biophoton emissions. As cells undergo metabolic processes stimulated by red light, they can potentially emit biophotons that facilitate communication and healing within the body. The enhanced cellular activity induced by red-light therapy might lead to a more organized emission of biophotons, suggesting improved cellular communication. Theories propose that red-light therapy can positively influence HRV, indicating improved autonomic nervous system function and better stress response. This was demonstrated in a clinical study involving 151 university students.[138] During a two-hour session, participants were monitored at rest and while participating in cognitively demanding tasks under two different lighting conditions—3500K white light (LED) and peak wavelengths in the near-infrared (875 nm, 960 nm) and far-red (735 nm) spectrum. The addition of the red-light spectrums positively improved resting high-frequency HRV, high-frequency HRV to cognitive demand, and feelings of pleasure. Interestingly, the red light also reduced performance on a visual search task. Altogether, these results reveal that red light spectrums are important for influencing humans at a psychological and physiological level, with implications for overall health.

By promoting relaxation and reducing inflammation, RLT can contribute to increased HRV, which is associated with enhanced overall health. The wavelengths of red and near-infrared light are believed to resonate with specific biological processes. Each color and wavelength interacts differently with biological tissues and can promote healing by improving cellular communication and energy production. Red-light therapy is thought to interact with the human biofield, potentially harmonizing energy flow within this field.

Scientists are discovering that low-intensity red and near-infrared light can affect cellular function. They believe this light interacts with a specific part of our cells called cytochrome c oxidase—the final enzyme in the electron transport chain of mitochondria that acts like a tiny engine in our cells that helps them efficiently produce energy. The light seems to help this engine work more efficiently, which can have positive effects on our bodies, like reducing inflammation and promoting healing. Interestingly, the light might work better when our cells are under stress. This suggests that people who are stressed or have certain health conditions might benefit more from this type of light therapy.

Light, as a fundamental manifestation of energy, interacts with living systems in profound ways. Each color in the light spectrum corresponds to a specific wavelength, frequency, and energy level, which can uniquely interact with the body and its subtle energy systems. The notion that specific light wavelengths or colors can influence divine energy is intriguing and deserves further exploration.

For instance, red light, with its longer wavelength and lower frequency, is associated with grounding and vitality. It stimulates mitochondrial activity, promoting energy production at a cellular level, which can be interpreted as amplifying divine energy to invigorate and sustain physical health. Blue light, on the other hand, with its shorter wavelength and higher frequency, is known for its calming effects. It influences circadian rhythms and melatonin production, aligning the body's natural cycles with divine harmony. Green light, positioned in the middle of the spectrum, is often seen as a balancing force. It fosters growth, renewal, and emotional equilibrium, aligning with the concept of divine energy as a source of healing and life-sustaining power. It harmonizes the body's energy flow, encouraging coherence and unity.

Rooted in Wellness: Harnessing Earth's Energy for Healing, Balance, and Restored Harmony

Earthing and grounding are terms often used interchangeably, but they refer to slightly different practices and contexts. Both concepts involve a connection to the Earth's electrical energy, which proponents claim can bring various health benefits. Earthing refers to the practice of direct physical contact with the Earth's surface (e.g., walking barefoot on grass, sand, or soil). This connection allows the body to absorb the Earth's electrons, which may neutralize free radicals and result in various health benefits. On the other hand, grounding typically refers to using technological methods designed to simulate the effects of earthing without direct physical contact with the Earth. This could include using grounding mats, sheets, or bands that are connected to the electrical grid or grounded to the Earth. It may seem peculiar that such a simple practice might benefit human health, but the mechanisms by which grounding and earthing work are grounded—pun intended— in scientific principles.

The Earth carries a negative charge, and direct contact with it can allow electrons to flow into the body, potentially promoting physiological benefits (e.g., improved sleep, reduced pain, enhanced mood). Through this exchange of energy, earthing may help stabilize the human biofield by aligning and balancing the body's energy with the Earth's energy, thus promoting overall harmony. Grounding has also been linked to a balancing effect on the autonomic nervous system, fostering a state of relaxation and coherence that supports overall health. From a spiritual perspective, grounding bonds the human body with the Earth's divine energy, reinforcing the interconnectedness between nature and well-being.

Grounding or earthing improves balance in sympathetic and parasympathetic nervous system function. Many people describe feeling a subtle energy shift or feeling more connected to nature when earthing or grounding. A sense of calm and relaxation is also frequently experienced. This may be a sign of changes in HRV, hormonal secretion, and coherence in nervous system function, all potential signs of enhanced divine energy utilization.

A double-blind clinical study evaluated the effects of grounding on human physiology in fifty-eight healthy adults.[139] Participants in the study were grounded to the earth by contact with a cord connected to a rod driven into the earth. Changes in brain and muscle activity were measured via electroencephalograms (EEG) and surface electromyograms (SEMGs). The researchers observed notable and sudden changes in the electrical activity of the participant's brains and muscles while grounding. Specifically, they saw a significant change in the left side of the brain, but not the right side. The observed changes in electrical activity provide evidence that grounding can induce physiological changes. They also saw a consistent and noteworthy change in the muscles in the upper back, on both sides. Reductions in blood volume pulse were noted in 86.4 percent of participants. Results of this study indicate that grounding may have a profound impact on neurological and muscular function, warranting further exploration into its potential therapeutic benefits for overall health.

Diurnal cortisol secretion levels, or the natural daily rhythm of cortisol production, play a significant role in sleep patterns and overall health. Cortisol levels normally follow a circadian rhythm, with levels peaking in the morning to help you wake up and gradually declining throughout the day, reaching their lowest point at night to promote sleep. When cortisol levels are disrupted, it can lead to various sleep problems, including waking up in the middle of the night. If cortisol levels remain elevated at night, it can interfere with the body's natural sleep-wake cycle, making it difficult to fall asleep and stay asleep. This can lead to fragmented sleep, poor sleep quality, and daytime fatigue. And as described earlier, chronically elevated cortisol levels can negatively affect overall health and increase the risk of chronic diseases.

A small clinical study measured the effects of grounding on cortisol levels during sleep.[140] Twelve participants who complained of sleep dysfunction, pain, and stress were grounded during sleep for eight weeks via a conductive mattress pad on their own beds. Cortisol levels were measured at four-hour intervals for a 24-hour period at baseline and again at six weeks after intervention. What the results showed was that connecting the body to the earth during sleep normalizes circadian cortisol profiles and reduces self-reported sleep dysfunction, pain, and stress.[141] Essentially, grounding reduced nighttime cortisol levels and resynchronized cortisol secretion to align with a healthy 24-hour circadian rhythm profile.

To rule out the placebo effect, another study compared grounding for two hours with sham grounding for the same amount of time.[142] An immediate decrease in skin conductance was observed while grounding but not in those who were in the sham grounding group. In fact, the sham group experienced the exact opposite, presenting with a noticeable and immediate increase in skin conductance. Skin conductance is a physiological measure of how well your skin conducts electricity. It's closely linked to the activity of the sympathetic nervous system, which controls the "fight-or-flight" response. Decreased skin conductance is linked to reduced arousal and stress, relaxation, and parasympathetic nervous system dominance (greater "rest-and-digest" activity). Additionally, respiratory rate variance increased, blood oxygenation variance decreased—followed by a dramatic increase after grounding, HRV increased, and perfusion index variance increased in the grounding group compared to controls. These findings are indicative of reduced stress and a heightened healing state.

Embracing Light, Sound, and the Earth's Anchoring Effect for Extraordinary Healing

In the intricate symphony of light, sound, and Earth's grounding embrace, we discover profound pathways to connect with divine energy for healing and balance. Each modality—whether through the illuminating power of light therapies, the harmonic resonance of sound, or the stabilizing effects of grounding—invites us to align with the universe's inherent vibrational order. The integration of advanced technologies like biofeedback and bioresonance further bridges the gap between science and spirituality, offering tools to measure, harmonize, and amplify this sacred connection. By embracing these practices, we empower ourselves to tap into the limitless potential of divine energy, fostering physical, emotional, and spiritual transformation. As we deepen our connection with these energies, we honor the innate wisdom within us and the universe, stepping into a state of coherence and healing that rises above the ordinary and welcomes the extraordinary.

CHAPTER NINE

The Influence of Natural Solutions on Divine Energy: Essential Oils and Dietary Supplements

The connection between nature and spirituality is as ancient as humanity itself, with countless traditions recognizing the healing power of the Earth's gifts. Natural remedies not only nourish the body but also elevate the spirit, harmonizing our physical and energetic being. Essential oils, with their potent aromatic compounds, and dietary supplements, rich in vital nutrients and bioactive compounds, have long been revered for their ability to align us with the divine energy that flows through all living things. Whether balancing energetic centers, amplifying the innate healing ability of the body, or deepening our connection to a higher power, essential oils and dietary supplements can unlock a path to holistic well-being.

Essential Oils: Multitarget, Multi-mechanism, Complex, and Potent Remedies for Health

Essential oils are the most potent natural remedies available and endowed with polypharmacology. As natural complex substances with from a dozen to hundreds of constituents, each with its own properties, they are multitarget, multi-mechanism solutions that possess inherent synergistic, additive, and antagonistic (or buffering) effects within a single essential oil. Each constituent in an essential oil possesses its own unique properties, cellular target binding potentials, and ability to interact with enzymes. Creating blends of two or more oils produces an even more complex chemistry and increases the potential to interact with proteins, enzymes, cellular targets, and biological pathways to maintain and restore optimum health.

Clinical research found that inhaling Douglas fir or lavender essential oil from a diffuser while performing an art activity balanced heart rate variability—low-frequency to high-frequency heart rate ratio, balancing autonomic nervous system activity and promoting relaxation.[143] Moreover, the oils decreased high beta brainwaves (indicating reduced stress), increased high alpha brainwaves (suggestive of a relaxed but focused state), and decreased gamma brainwaves (corresponding to a more relaxed state). A balanced autonomic nervous system is crucial for overall health and well-being, ensuring that the body can effectively respond to both stress and relaxation. Inhaled essential oils quickly travel to the brain and trigger neuroendocrine responses that could explain these changes, but a direct interaction with divine energy cannot be ruled out.

Taking an exam can be a stressful event that dysregulates cardiovascular and nervous system function. Russian scientists evaluated the effects of inhaling orange essential oil on HRV in students taking an exam.[144] Inhalation of the oil corrected indices of HRV, stabilizing psychophysiological state. By normalizing HRV, the oil shifted participants to a more relaxed state, potentially improving focus and reducing anxiety. This research provides evidence that inhaling orange essential oil may be a simple and accessible method for reducing exam stress and promoting a more balanced physiological state.

Workplace stress is also challenging, especially if you have a high-stress occupation or a stress-provoking supervisor. Inhalation of bergamot essential oil was assessed in elementary school teachers in Taiwan.[145] Inhaling the oil for ten minutes produced rapid and significant increases in HRV and high-frequency power percentage, again suggesting coherence was achieved through essential oil inhalation. These findings suggest that bergamot essential oil inhalation may be a simple and effective strategy for managing workplace stress among educators and potentially other professionals in high-stress environments.

The majority of women experience some degree of uncomfortable symptoms immediately preceding and during menstruation. A clinical study determined that inhaling yuzu essential oil for only ten minutes significantly decreased heart rate and increased high-frequency power of HRV, reflecting balanced parasympathetic nervous system activity, during the luteal phase.[146] Tension-anxiety, anger-hostility, total mood disturbance, and fatigue were all improved as well. The psychoneurophysiologic effects of yuzu were considered comparable to lavender oil, which was used as a positive control in the study. These promising results suggest that incorporating yuzu essential oil into premenstrual care routines could offer a natural and effective means of alleviating distressing symptoms, providing women with a valuable alternative alongside traditional remedies.

Another inhalation study demonstrated that inhaling eucalyptus essential oil with menthol (the primary constituent of quality peppermint oil) increased heart rate variability, improved pain tolerance, and enhanced blood oxygenation.[147] Specifically, participants reported enhanced physiological responses, indicating better autonomic regulation and comfort levels in high-temperature settings, thereby suggesting that inhaling essential oils can have beneficial effects on stress responses and overall well-being during exposure to heat. Each of these studies serves as emerging evidence that inhaling essential oils can balance autonomic nervous system function and increase resilience to stress. They also show that delivering essential oils to the olfactory system has strong physiological effects across a number of bodily functions.

Inhalation isn't the only way to enjoy, or leverage, the profound effects of essential oils. Researchers compared the outcome after applying a placebo cosmetic product or one enriched with essential oils.[148] The enriched topical product consisted of Phoenician juniper gum extract, copaiba resin, rosewood essential oil, and Virginia cedarwood essential oil. The placebo and enriched oil products were applied by participants for 28 days. The essential oil-based product dampened cortisol increases triggered by a psychosocial stress test, reduced anxiety, favorably improved mood, and reduced nonverbal behavior patterns indicative of anxiety, motivational conflict, and avoidance. The overall outcome was improved stress resilience, which was attributed to positive effects on physiological parameters as well as the neuroendocrine and psychological systems.

The effects of essential oils on the human biofield in young healthy individuals has also been assessed.[149] The body's energy biofield was recorded by PIP biofield imaging system before and after inhalation of tagetes, frankincense, lilac, French basil, rosemary, and palmarosa essential oils. Remarkable changes in the participants' biofields were seen after inhaling the essential oils. Lilac, basil, and rosemary each reduced biofield green colors and markedly increased biofield yellow colors around the head, indicating soothing and relaxing effects. Palmarosa increased green and reduced yellow colors in the biofield, suggesting increased vibrational frequency, elevated mood, and an aroused and refreshed state. Frankincense significantly reduced yellow around the head similarly to palmarosa, but didn't appear to affect green colors. This is very interesting, since this type of effect may indicate emotional distress, challenges in engaging in social interactions, a lack of focus, or a diminished sense of happiness. One way to interpret these results is that frankincense might be facilitating the release of negative energies or emotional blockages associated with qualities represented by the yellow color—such as mental clarity, joy, and effective communication. Only mild changes were observed when inhaling tagetes. All of this suggests that essential oils interact with the human biofield and produce profound changes that can improve health.

Due to their small size and molecular weight, essential oils are ideal solutions to cross the blood-brain barrier (BBB) and positively influence brain structure, activity, or function. The BBB is a selective permeability barrier that protects the brain from potentially harmful substances while allowing certain small molecules to pass through. Many essential oils contain compounds such as terpenes, phenols, and esters, which can have neuroprotective effects. For example, the chemical constituents of lavender and rosemary have been shown to influence neurotransmitter systems—like serotonin and dopamine—leading to improved mood, reduced anxiety, and enhanced cognitive function.[150,151,152] Certain essential oils may promote neurogenesis or improve synaptic plasticity, contributing to a more adaptable neural network.[153,154] This can potentially enhance cognitive functions such as memory, learning, and emotional regulation. The fragrant properties of essential oils may have a profound impact on mood and emotional state.[155,156,157] By elevating one's mood or creating a sense of calm and clarity, individuals may find it easier to connect with higher states of consciousness or spiritual guidance. It is possible that these alterations in brain structure and function can lead to enhanced connection to divine energy.

A clinical study consisting of fifty women (twenty-eight rose intervention group and twenty-two control) aged 41 to 69 evaluated the brain effects of continuous inhalation of rose essential oil.[158] Participants wore a patch containing one to three drops of a 0.5% dilution of rose essential oil or water daily on their clothes for one month. Brain effects were measured using magnetic resonance imaging. Remarkably, continuous inhalation of rose essential oil increased gray matter volume in the whole brain and posterior cingulate cortex, which suggests inhaling rose oil could shield against brain atrophy and cognitive decline. That such a simple intervention could produce positive structural changes to the brain is mind-boggling, unless you know how unique and matchless essential oils are.

Gray matter refers to the brain tissue rich in neural cell bodies, dendrites, and synapses. Increased gray matter can be associated with improved cognitive functions, such as memory, attention, and processing speed. Some theories propose that increased gray matter might be linked to enhanced consciousness, self-awareness, or even spiritual experiences. Could this increased gray matter designate a greater connection to divine energy or a more vivid sense of spiritual experiences? The thought that increased gray matter may be linked to divine energy offers intriguing possibilities for exploring this idea using various theoretical frameworks.

Research suggests that deterioration of olfaction (sense of smell) precedes a decline in cognitive abilities.[159] Indeed, olfactory loss is associated with significant losses of brain matter (gray and white) in humans. Loss of olfaction can even predict the progression of mild cognitive impairment to Alzheimer's disease.

Knowing the correlation between olfaction and cognition, researchers set out to investigate whether olfactory enrichment (exposure to pleasant fragrances) could improve memory in older adults (aged 60 to 85 years)..[160] Participants in the study were provided a diffuser and seven essential oils as fragrances (rose, orange, eucalyptus, lemon, peppermint, rosemary, and lavender). Participants diffused each oil for two hours as they slept in a rotating manner—changing the oil they diffused each night. This process was continued for six months. The researchers found that fragrances have privileged access to areas of the brain and pathways relevant to olfaction and memory, which may help normalize brain circuitry linked to memory function. Remarkably, nightly diffusion improved cognition, memory, and neural functioning by 226%! They also found that olfactory enrichment increased the volume of the uncinate fasciculus, a white matter tract that connects the hippocampus and the prefrontal cortex. Increases in this area of the brain are associated with better language skills, improved cognitive flexibility, and enhanced creativity. The uncinate fasciculus also plays a critical role in integrating emotional experiences with cognitive processes. Increases in the uncinate fasciculus might also be seen as a mechanism for enhancing consciousness and its influence on the quantum realm. Consciousness may operate on a quantum level, with phenomena such as entanglement and coherence potentially playing a role. If consciousness arises from quantum processes, then any neuroanatomical changes in structures such as the uncinate fasciculus that enhance emotional cognition could potentially deepen one's connection to these quantum states. This study suggests that olfactory enrichment may be a promising new way to not only improve memory in older adults but also channel divine energy.

While limited scientific evidence exists regarding how essential oils interact with the human biofield, change vibrational frequency, or alter biophoton emission because few researchers have explored this connection, the possibility that essential oils are working with divine energy to promote healing is fascinating. The fact that chemistry and the physical properties of essential oils are directly associated with their therapeutic activity does not rule out that this chemistry, also fashioned by God, is intermingled with divine energy.

Herbal Wisdom and Modern Science: The Evolution of Dietary Supplements and Nutraceuticals for Enhanced Health and Consciousness

Herbs and plants have been used as medicines for thousands of years, dating back to ancient civilizations such as Egypt, Greece, and China. These early cultures recognized the medicinal properties of plants and developed traditional medicine practices that relied heavily on herbal remedies. Many traditional medicines still used today, such as willow bark for pain relief and foxglove for heart conditions, originated from ancient herbal practices. Traditional knowledge, honed through generations of trial and error, is now being substantiated by modern scientific research, which is elucidating the underlying mechanisms and pathways of these remedies.

As modern medicine developed, herbal remedies were adapted into dietary supplements and nutraceuticals. Dietary supplements are products that contain one or more dietary ingredients, such as vitamins, minerals, herbs, or amino acids, that are intended to supplement the diet. Nutraceuticals are a subset of dietary supplements that contain naturally occurring ingredients and compounds that have pharmacologic effects in mitigating health conditions.

The 1960s saw the rise of modern herbalism, with the establishment of the formal herbal medicine schools and the development of standardized herbal products. Pioneers like Nicholas Culpeper, Dr. John Christopher, and David Hoffmann are key contributors to the revival of herbalism. Nutraceuticals trended in the 1990s as active compounds were identified and purified. Advances in technology and manufacturing have enabled the creation of high-quality dietary supplements and nutraceuticals with consistent potency and purity. Modern adaptations have led to the development of more effective dietary supplements and nutraceuticals, which have become a significant part of the healthcare landscape, and millions of people rely on them for good health.

Since many supplements and nutraceuticals are derived from natural sources, they inherently contain the same divine energy by which humans were created and therefore harmoniously work with our own healing divine energy. One of the most common supplements taken in the modern era is a multinutrient that provides vitamins and minerals often deficient in modern foods.

Over the years, modern farming practices have prioritized traits like size, yield, taste, and shelf life. This focus has often come at the expense of nutritional value. Globally, it is estimated that approximately 4 to 5 billion people get insufficient amounts of key nutrients from their diet. Insufficient levels of iodine (68 percent of the population), vitamin E (67 percent of the population), calcium (66 percent of the population), iron (65 percent of the population), riboflavin (55 percent of the population), folate (54 percent of the population), and vitamin C (53 percent of the population) are reported in research.[161] Inadequate intakes of vitamin B12, selenium, magnesium, zinc, vitamin A, thiamin, and niacin were also noted. That means most of us are not getting the daily nutrients our bodies need to function optimally.

Based on inadequate intake of these key micronutrients, it is highly plausible that most of us are deficient or have insufficient levels of at least one micronutrient, likely multiple micronutrients. Without the ideal level of micronutrients, we can experience a range of short-term and long-term health problems, such as fatigue and weakness, poor immune function, hair loss, digestive issues, skin problems, heart disease, cancer, diabetes, osteoporosis, neurological disorders, and developmental delays in children. It is clear that taking a daily multinutrient is a crucial key to good health and health span.

French researchers conducted a study that aimed to assess the effects of a daily multinutrient with guarana on cognitive performance and HRV.[162] They compared the effects to a caffeine supplement and placebo. Fifty-six subjects participated in a randomized, double-blind crossover study, consisting of three experimental sessions conducted on different days. Cognitive performance and HRV were assessed 15 minutes prior to taking the multinutrient, 15 minutes after taking the multinutrient, and then again every 15 minutes for three hours. Cognitive responsiveness was faster—without affecting accuracy—30 and 90 minutes after taking the multinutrient. HRV decreased during the first hour in participants who took the placebo and caffeine supplement, while HRV remained stable among those who took the multinutrient. Altogether, the findings suggest that taking this multinutrient with guarana stabilizes autonomic nervous system regulation (coherence) and enhances decision-making performance.

A review of cross-sectional and interventional studies examined the relationship between HRV and micronutrients.[163] Due to the scant research available and the significant differences in study methodologies, populations, and outcomes, a definitive link between HRV and micronutrients could not be made. However, the accumulating evidence suggests that deficiencies in vitamins D and B12 are associated with reduced HRV. Additionally, zinc supplementation during pregnancy had positive effects on the

HRV of offspring up until age 5. Given the positive trend indicating a link between micronutrient status and HRV, HRV may be an objective way to validate the benefits of dietary supplements and nutraceuticals.

Most parents strive to do all they can to provide a high-quality life for their children, including emphasizing proactive measures to improve health. However, few realize how their daily choices today can affect their future offspring. Going back to the topic of epigenetics, what we experience, such as diet, stress, and exposure to toxins, can affect how our genes work. These epigenetic changes can be passed down to future generations, influencing their health and development. Studies have shown that the diet of pregnant mothers can affect the health of their children and even grandchildren due to a process known as epigenetic inheritance.[164, 165, 166] A mother's diet can influence the development of her child's metabolic programming and their risk of developing certain diseases like obesity, diabetes, and heart disease. An animal model found that feeding mice a low-protein diet affected their offspring for four generations.[167] These next generations had lower birth weights and smaller kidneys, putting them at greater risk of chronic kidney disease and high blood pressure. These inherited epigenetic changes can then influence the gene expression of future generations. Similarly, a father's lifestyle choices, such as smoking or exposure to toxins, can also impact the health of his offspring.[168, 169, 170] Parental choices can have a profound impact on the health and well-being of their children and future generations through epigenetic mechanisms alone. You are what you eat then becomes a mantra for not only you, but your future kids and grandkids as well.

MTHFR (Methylenetetrahydrofolate reductase) is a gene that provides instructions for making an enzyme involved in the metabolism of homocysteine. Homocysteine is an amino acid in the blood that, at elevated levels, is associated with an increased risk of cardiovascular disease and other health issues. When this gene has certain variations or mutations, it can impair the body's ability to process homocysteine, leading to elevated levels. Vitamin B12 plays a crucial role in the metabolism of homocysteine. It works in conjunction with folate to convert homocysteine into methionine, a vital amino acid for protein synthesis, methylation, gene regulation, DNA repair, neurotransmitter synthesis, nutrient absorption, detoxification, and antioxidant function. When individuals have MTHFR mutations, their bodies may struggle to efficiently utilize vitamin B12. This can lead to a functional deficiency of B12, even if blood levels appear normal. So, even though there's plenty of vitamin B12 in the body, it's not being used properly. It's like having a full tank of gas but none of it is getting to the engine to start the car.

The most crucial developmental period for the human central nervous system is gestation. Vitamin B12 deficiency in pregnant mothers increases the occurrence of neurological deficits in their offspring. Researchers evaluated the effects of low maternal vitamin B12 status during pregnancy and its effects on heart function regulation by the autonomic nervous system in their offspring.[171] The primary measurement of this activity was HRV and frequency domain. There was a significant correlation between low-frequency and total power HRV and cord blood vitamin B12 levels. Children born to mothers with lower vitamin D levels had reduced control of heart function (heart rate, blood pressure, contractility) by the sympathetic nervous system. Potentially, this could lead to long-term poor ability to enhance HRV in these children.

As mentioned previously, BDNF is a protein that plays a crucial role in brain health and function. It directly influences brain energy metabolism and neuroplasticity. A clinical study concluded that 12 weeks of zinc gluconate supplementation decreased depression in overweight and obese individuals.[172] Further investigation discovered that zinc supplementation significantly increased BDNF levels in the blood. Another nutraceutical that affects BDNF levels is turmeric, which is nearly always standardized to curcuminoids. Males aged 31 to 59 years with major depressive disorder were randomly assigned to receive 1,000 mg of curcumin or a soybean placebo daily for six weeks.[173] Not only did the curcumin reduce depression and inflammatory markers (cytokines interleukin 1β and tumor necrosis factor α), it also increased BDNF levels and simultaneously reduced cortisol levels. An increase in BDNF suggests greater neuroplasticity could imply accessing divine energy to facilitate healing, akin to neuroplasticity's role in recovery and adaptation.

The connection between the gut microbiome, probiotic supplementation, and BDNF is an area of growing interest in both neuroscience and nutritional science. The gut microbiome refers to the diverse community of microorganisms, including bacteria, fungi, viruses, and protozoa, that reside in the gastrointestinal tract. These microorganisms play crucial roles in digestion, metabolism, immune function, and overall health. Research shows that the gut microbiome can influence the brain and behavior through various mechanisms, including the production of neurotransmitters, modulation of the immune system, and interaction with the vagus nerve (which connects the gut and brain). Some studies suggest that specific probiotics may enhance the production of BDNF in the brain, leading to improved mood, cognitive function, and resilience against stress.

A randomized, double-blind, and placebo-controlled clinical trial sought to determine if supplementing with probiotics containing *Bifidobacterium bifidum* BGN4 and *Bifidobacterium longum* BORI for twelve weeks would affect cognitive function and mood in older adults.[174] The sixty-three participants were randomly assigned to take probiotics or a placebo and both the gut microbiome and cognitive function were assessed. At the end of the study, a positive shift in the gut microbiome (decrease in relative abundance of inflammation-producing gut bacteria) and marked increases in BDNF levels were observed. Participants also experienced improved cognitive flexibility and decreased stress. A separate study compared the effects of a synbiotic (probiotics plus prebiotics) containing *Lactobacillus acidophilus* T16, *Bifidobacterium bifidum* BIA-6, *Bifidobacterium lactis* BIA-7, and *Bifidobacterium longum* BIA-8 or a probiotic with the same strains and maltodextrin instead of prebiotics.[175] The population consisted of seventy-five people undergoing hemodialysis—a medical procedure that uses a machine to filter and remove waste products and excess fluids from the blood when the kidneys are unable to perform this function adequately. After twelve weeks of supplementation, a subgroup of participants in the synbiotic group showed significant increases in BDNF. In general, the synbiotic group had greater improvement in depression and BDNF levels compared to the probiotic-only group.

Harmonizing with the Divine: Unlocking Healing and Potential Through Natural Solutions

The influence of natural solutions, including dietary supplements and nutraceuticals, on divine energy underscores the profound connection between creation and Creator. Nutraceuticals and dietary supplements are not merely tools for physical well-being; they are gifts designed to enhance our capacity to align with divine energy and fulfill our God-given potential. By embracing these natural solutions with gratitude and stewardship, we unlock the ability to heal, restore, and elevate body, mind, emotions, and spirit. As we apply these principles in our daily lives, we not only honor the Creator's design but also become instruments of His love and power, amplifying the flow of divine energy within ourselves and the world around us.

REFLEXOLOGY FOOT/ANKLE CHART
Part 1

0 Hypophysis (pituitary)
1 Head
2 Frontal sinuses
3 Brainstem, cerebellum
4 Epiphysis
5 Temple, trigeminal
6 Nose
7 Nape
8 Eyes
9 Ears
10 Shoulder
11 Trapezium
12 Thyroid
13 Parathyroid
14 Lungs, bronchus
15 Stomach
16 Duodenum
17 Pancreas
18 Liver
19 Gall bladder
20 Solar plexus
21 Suprarenal
22 Kidney
23 Ureter
24 Urinary bladder
25 Intestinum tenue
26 Appendix
27 Ileoceleal valve
28 Ascending colon
29 colon transversum
30 Descending colon
31 Intestinum rectum
32 Anus
33 Heart and blood circulation
34 Spleen
35 Knee
36 Ovary, Falloppian tube/testicles
37 Underbelly
38 Hip
39 Lymph nodes (head, Thorax, armpits)
40 Lymph nodes (Abdomen)
41 Tanker lymphatic (Thorax, trachea)
42 Inner ear (balance)
43 Breast / Chest
44 Diaphragm
45 Tonsils
46 Maximilar lower
47 Maximilar top
48 Larynx, trachea
49 Anus
50 Uterus / Prostate
51 Vagina / Penis, urethra
52 Bowel straight Hemorrhoids
53 Cervical vertebrae
54 Thoracic vertebrae
55 Lumbar vertebrae
56 Sacral and cixigeas

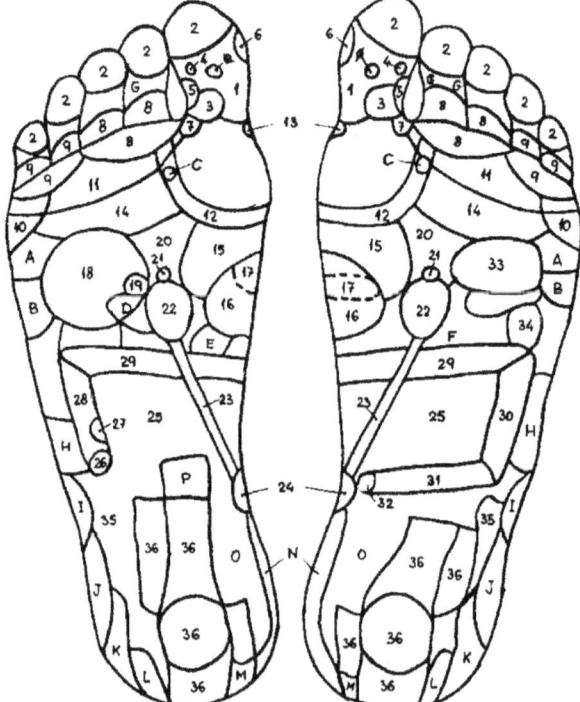

CHAPTER TEN

Harness Divine Energy and Be Healthy

The culmination of this journey through divine energy and its transformative power brings us to a profound realization: the interplay between the divine and the physical is not only the essence of healing but also the gateway to restoring harmony within ourselves and the world around us. As His children earnestly seek Him and exercise faith in Jesus Christ, God manifests miraculous ways to employ divine energy to heal all things, including the Earth itself. Advancement in human healing must emphasize ways to continuously hone our ability to harness divine energy and integrate it into every aspect of our lives.

The Divine Blueprint: A Perfect and Infinite Body

In its perfect state, the human body reflects divine design—flawless and infinite, capable of extraordinary resilience and eternal renewal. Yet, the effects of mortality—brought on by the fall of Adam and Eve, environmental stressors, and spiritual disconnection—can obscure this perfection. The process of healing, therefore, is not merely about treating symptoms but about aligning with the divine blueprint embedded within us. This alignment is facilitated through a harmonious interplay of physical, energetic, and spiritual dimensions.

When we consider manifestations like HRV, biophoton emission, the human biofield, and neuroplasticity, we see glimpses of this divine design in measurable terms. HRV reflects the adaptability and resilience of our autonomic nervous system, serving as a mirror to our physical and emotional well-being. Biophoton emission reveals the light energy emitted by our cells, a testament to the body's inherent vitality. The human biofield, encompassing vibrational frequencies, demonstrates the electromagnetic energy that radiates from us, echoing the unseen yet palpable connection to divine energy. Neuroplasticity enables individuals to reshape their neural pathways and consciousness, fostering a profound sense of unity with God and enhancing their spiritual connection and understanding.

These measurable phenomena are not merely clinical data points; they are evidence of a higher order. They demonstrate that as we seek to align our physical and spiritual selves, we unlock greater potential for healing and wholeness.

The Inseparable Nature of the Body and Spirit

The body and spirit are intrinsically linked, each influencing the other in a complex dance of life. They are inseparable due to their profound interdependence and the holistic nature of human existence. The body serves as the physical vessel through which the spirit experiences and interacts with the world. Every thought, emotion, and spiritual insight manifests through physical sensations and actions. Our bodily states influence our spiritual states, and vice versa—emotional or spiritual distress can manifest in physical symptoms, highlighting the unity between the two. We must fervently endeavor to maintain a healthy vessel (body) for our spirit to unite with divine energy.

Both the body and spirit are composed of divine energy, or the Light of Christ. Energetic systems illustrate how our physical form and spiritual essence are interconnected. This energy flows through us, and when one aspect is imbalanced or blocked, it can affect the other, reinforcing the idea that we are holistic beings. Acknowledging the inseparability of body and spirit encourages a holistic approach to health, integrating physical, emotional, mental, and spiritual facets of well-being. This perspective fosters greater self-awareness, self-care, and healing practices that nurture both the physical body and the spiritual essence, promoting overall harmony and balance.

Daily Practices: Honing Our Ability to Harness Divine Energy

The path toward mastering the use of divine energy for healing is both sacred and practical. It demands consistency, intentionality, and faith. Daily practices are the crucible in which this mastery is forged. By incorporating energy healing techniques, sound therapy, light therapy, essential oils, dietary supplements, nutrition, and exercise into our routines, we lay the groundwork for a life attuned to divine energy. Consistency is key!

Energy healing techniques harness the vibrational essence of our being, facilitating alignment with the divine flow of cosmic energy. Modalities such as Reiki and healing touch create pathways for life force energy to circulate freely, dissolving obstacles that inhibit our spiritual and emotional wellness. The gentle touch of hands, guided by intention, acts as a conduit for divine energy, promoting profound healing and restoring balance. Incorporating mindfulness practices enhances our attunement to this energy, allowing for a deeper connection with the Creator's love and wisdom. By embracing these sacred techniques, we not only invite healing but also embody the divine resonance that exists within and around us, manifesting our highest potential.

Resonant frequencies have the power to align our energetic centers, dissolve emotional obstructions, and restore harmony. Using tools like tuning forks, singing bowls, or even inspired music, we can attune our bodies to frequencies that resonate with divine order. These sound vibrations penetrate our cells and tissues, creating a therapeutic environment where healing can flourish, allowing us to access deeper states of consciousness and expand our spiritual awareness. By consciously engaging with these frequencies, we can cultivate an inner landscape of peace and balance, inviting the divine to flow through us more abundantly.

From the sun's natural rays to targeted photobiomodulation devices, light provides a profound stimulus for cellular repair and energy production. It reminds us of the divine declaration: "Let there be light," a command that continues to sustain life and healing. This radiant energy not only penetrates our physical form but also nourishes our spirit, illuminating hidden aspects of our consciousness that yearn for recognition and healing. By embracing various light therapies, we open ourselves to an empowering experience that uplifts our vibrational frequency and aligns us with the greater cosmic symphony of creation.

Incorporating relaxation techniques such as meditation and deep breathing helps to quiet the mind and open the heart to divine energy. Meditation, in particular, serves as a bridge between the spiritual and physical, fostering inner peace and enhancing the body's capacity for renewal. These practices reduce stress, balance the biofield, and prepare the body to receive healing energy, allowing us to become more receptive to divine insights and guidance. As we cultivate this inner stillness, we not only enhance our personal well-being but also tap into a collective consciousness that connects us to all beings.

The aromatic compounds of plants carry vibrational energy that interacts with our physiology and biofield. Oils such as frankincense and lavender are not only tools for relaxation but also for enhancing transcendent clarity and connection. When inhaled, applied, or ingested, essential oils can trigger profound emotional releases and elevate our vibrational state, creating an inviting atmosphere for richer connection with divine energy. Their ancient use in sacred rituals embodies a deep wisdom that reminds us of the Earth's ability to nurture and heal, reinforcing our bond with nature and the divine.

The incorporation of dietary supplements and nutraceuticals into our daily routines serves as an essential complement to our holistic health journey. These supplements, derived from natural sources, bridge the gap between nutrition and wellness, providing targeted support to enhance our energetic and physical well-being. Just as we seek to align with divine energy through meditation and movement, nourishing our bodies with the right vitamins, minerals, and botanical extracts can optimize cellular function and elevate our vibrational states. For instance, adaptogens like ashwagandha and rhodiola can help mitigate stress and foster resilience, enabling us to remain attuned to the flow of divine energy. By consciously integrating these supplements into our lifestyle, we fortify our sacred vessels, ensuring they are equipped to channel the healing forces of the universe effectively. This mindful approach to nutrition not only supports our physical health but also deepens our connection to the divine, promoting an overall sense of balance, vitality, and spiritual clarity. Through this synergy of dietary awareness and energetic practices, we cultivate an elevated state of being where the divine energy can flow through us more freely, allowing us to manifest our highest potential.

Nourishing the body with what it needs to thrive is a foundational act of stewardship. Whole foods and supplements rich in essential nutrients fortify the body's natural defenses and amplify its ability to channel divine energy. By consciously choosing nourishing foods, we honor our sacred vessel and create a strong foundation for spiritual practices, enabling us to better embody our true essence. As we cultivate a holistic approach to nourishment, we grow in awareness of the interconnectedness of body, mind, and spirit, enhancing our capacity to receive and express divine love.

Movement is a form of worship that acknowledges the gift of life, health, and existence. It not only strengthens the body but also aligns us with the rhythmic flow of life. Exercise stimulates neuroplasticity, enhances HRV, and supports overall vitality, enabling us to better receive and utilize divine energy. Whether through dance, aerobics, strength training, or simply walking in nature, each motion becomes an offering, a celebration of the divine presence within us. As we engage in these physical expressions, we release stagnant energy and invite a fluid connection to the universe, harmonizing our physical form with our spiritual essence.

The Role of Neuroplasticity in Divine Healing

The brain's capacity for change, or neuroplasticity, is a striking example of divine ingenuity. This inherent ability allows us to rewire neural pathways through intentional practices such as positive habits, faith-based affirmations, and purposeful meditation, leading to profound healing and spiritual development. Engaging in these practices is not merely a psychological exercise; it represents a divine act of creation unfolding within us.

As we consciously direct our thoughts and intentions, we cultivate a fertile ground for growth, enabling the mind to evolve in alignment with our highest values and beliefs. The assertion that "as we think, so we become" encapsulates this dynamic, revealing the profound power of our thoughts to shape our identities and destinies. By aligning our cognitive processes with eternal truths—whether through scripture, spiritual principles, or truth declarations—we harness the life-changing potential inherent in neuroplasticity.

Each moment spent in reflection and mindful intention becomes an opportunity to not only heal past wounds but also to forge a new reality characterized by hope, resilience, and spiritual enlightenment, showcasing the extraordinary interplay between our cognitive faculties and the divine blueprint that guides our lives. This ongoing renewal journey exemplifies the synergy of science and spirituality, inviting us to embrace our creative power and align our mental landscapes with the divine, ultimately fostering a more profound experience of life.

Faith and the Miraculous

Faith is the catalyst that activates divine energy. It bridges the gap between the seen and unseen, allowing us to tap into God's infinite and omnipresent power. Through faith, we are not passive recipients but active participants in the healing process. When we sincerely seek Him with earnest hearts and unwavering trust, miracles become possible. These miracles may manifest in physical healing, emotional restoration, or even the healing of relationships and communities.

The scriptures remind us that faith the size of a mustard seed can move mountains. Similarly, even the smallest step toward exercising faith in Jesus Christ invites divine intervention. The miraculous becomes a natural outcome when divine energy flows unimpeded through our lives. Our power to wield divine energy increases as we exercise more faith in Jesus Christ. Break the cycle of doubt rehearsed in our minds, and become one with divine energy.

Healing the Earth Through Divine Energy

As stewards of God's creation, we are called to extend the principles of healing beyond ourselves to the world around us.

The Earth, in its perfect state, reflects divine glory—a flawless and infinite system designed to sustain life. Yet, just as the human body can become misaligned, so too can the Earth. Pollution, deforestation, and other forms of environmental degradation disrupt the Earth's natural rhythms.

Through intentional practices such as sustainable living, regenerative agriculture, and mindful consumption, we can participate in the healing of the Earth. These efforts are not merely ecological; they are spiritual acts of worship and alignment with divine will. The same divine energy that heals our bodies can restore balance to the Earth, making it a place of abundance and peace once more.

The Infinite Potential of Divine Energy

The journey to harness divine energy is ongoing, a testament to the infinite nature of both the Creator and His creation. Each day offers opportunities to refine our abilities, deepen our faith, and expand our understanding. We must maintain a heart receptive to divine energy and regularly focus its healing powers on cells, tissues, and organs. As we engage in this process, we discover that the limits we once perceived are but illusions. The body's potential for healing, renewal, and growth is boundless when aligned with and fostered by divine energy.

Deep within every soul lies a longing for connection—a yearning to feel seen, heard, known, and valued. Ultimately, we want to belong, and the most profound and transformative connection is with Jesus Christ. As we come unto Him and become more like Him, we begin to align with the divine order, harmonizing our lives with the eternal flow of divine energy. This connection goes beyond the superficial, reaching into the depths of our being to restore, uplift, and empower. Through Christ, we are not only reconnected to our Creator but also to the infinite love, peace, and purpose that flow from His divine nature. The closer we walk with Him, the more we reflect His Light, becoming conduits of healing and wholeness to ourselves and the world around us.

The integration of measurable tools like HRV, biophoton emission, and the biofield with practices such as sound therapy, light therapy, and mindful living provides a roadmap for accessing divine energy. However, it is faith that transforms this roadmap into a living journey. As we seek Him and align our lives with His will, we become conduits of His infinite power—not only for our own healing but for the healing of all creation. The invitation is clear: embrace this divine energy, live in harmony with its principles, and witness the miraculous unfold in every aspect of life. In this sacred dance between faith and practice, we awaken to the truth that our willingness to embody divine energy not only transforms our own existence but also illuminates the path for others, revealing that in the interconnected web of life, each act of love and healing reverberates through the cosmos, echoing the profound divine purpose we are all destined to fulfill.

REFLEXOLOGY FOOT/ANKLE CHART
Part 2

A - Clavicle
B - Sternum
C - Thymus
D - Pleura
E - Childbirth"
F - Ribs
G - Mouth
H - Lliaco
I - Thigh
J - Knee
K - Leg
L - Feet
M - Coccyx
N - Sacro
O - Hypogastric plexus
P - iliacus
Q - Sciatic nerve

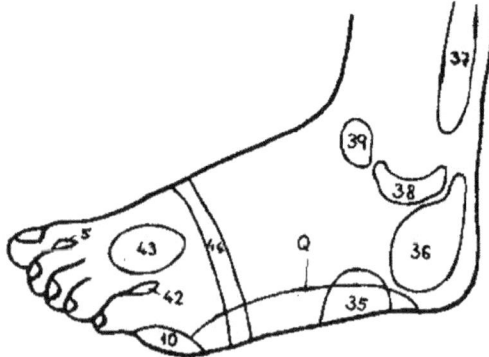

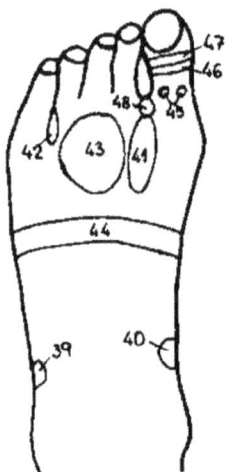

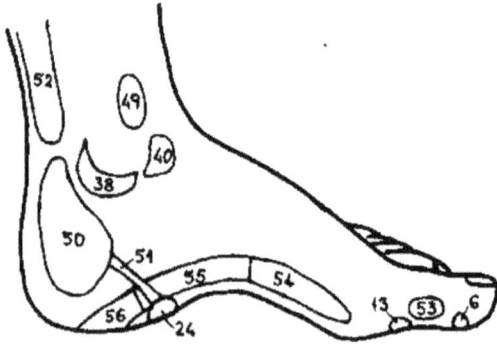

References

[1] Colloca L. The Fascinating Mechanisms and Implications of the Placebo Effect. *Int Rev Neurobiol.* 2018;138:xv–xx.

[2] Tilburt JC, Emanuel EJ, Kaptchuk TJ, et al. Prescribing "placebo treatments": results of national survey of US internists and rheumatologists. *BMJ.* 2008;337:a1938.

[3] Klinger R, Blasini M, Schmitz J, et al. Nocebo effects in clinical studies: hints for pain therapy. *Pain Rep.* 2017 Mar 15;2(2):e586.

[4] Cadossi R, Massari L, Racine-Avila J, et al. Pulsed Electromagnetic Field Stimulation of Bone Healing and Joint Preservation: Cellular Mechanisms of Skeletal Response. *J Am Acad Orthop Surg Glob Res Rev.* 2020 May 18;4(5):e19.00155.

[5] Thomas AW, Graham K, Prato FS, et al. A randomized, double-blind, placebo-controlled clinical trial using a low-frequency magnetic field in the treatment of musculoskeletal chronic pain. *Pain Res Manag.* 2007 Winter;12(4):249–258.

[6] Li M, Yao X, Sun L, et al. Effects of Electroconvulsive Therapy on Depression and Its Potential Mechanism. *Front Psychol.* 2020 Feb 20;11:80.

[7] Vance CGT, Dailey DL, Rakel BA, et al. Using TENS for pain control: the state of the evidence. *Pain Manag.* 2014 May;4(3):197–209.

[8] Rubik B. The Biofield Hypothesis: Its Biophysical Basis and Role in Medicine. *J Altern Complement Med.* 2003 Jan;8(6):703-17.

[9] Korotkov K. Measuring Human Energy Field Revolutionary Instrument to reveal Energy Fields of Human and Nature. Accessed from https://www.bio-well.com/assets/files/papers/BioEnergy/2013%20Measuring%20Energy%20Fields.pdf on 12-9-2024.

[10] McCraty R, Atkinson M, Bradley RT. Electrophysiological evidence of intuition: Part 2. A system-wide process? *J Altern Complement Med.* 2004;10(2):325-36.

[11] McCraty R, Atkinson M, Tomasino D, et al. The Electricity of Touch: Detection and measurement of cardiac energy exchange between people. Available at: http://www.abiomac.org.br/aartigos/ABIOMAC_1%20-%20Pesquisa%20-%20A%20eletricidade%20do%20toque%20-electricity-of-touch.pdf.

[12] McCarty R. The Energetic Heart: Biolectromagnetic Interactions Within and Between People. Available at: https://www.researchgate.net/publication/274451622_The_Energetic_Heart_Biolectromagnetic_Interactions_Within_and_Between_People.

[13] Nagoski A. *Burnout.* (2019). Avery Publishing.

[14] Alshami AM. Pain: Is It All in the Brain or the Heart? *Curr Pain Headache Rep.* 2019 Nov 14;23(12):88.

[15] Armour JA. Cardiac neuronal hierarchy in health and disease. *Am J Physiol.* 2004;287:R262–R271.

[16] Hashim AT, Albayati AS, Nazal E. Heart Memory and Feelings. *Springer Nature Link.* 2023 Jan 12:305-9.

[17] Tendulkar M, Tendulkar R, Dhanda PS, et al. Clinical potential of sensory neurites in the heart and their role in decision-making. *Front Neurosci.* 2024 Feb 13;17:1308232.

[18] Hasan W. Autonomic cardiac innervation. *Organogenesis.* 2013 May 14;9(3):176–193.

[19] Koza Y, Aydin MD, Bayram E, et al. The Role of Cardiac Ganglia in the Prevention of Coronary Atherosclerosis: An Analytical Examination of Cholesterol-fed Rabbits. *Balkan Med J.* 2020 Feb 28;37(2):79–83.

[20] Campos ID, Pinto V, Sousa N, et al. A brain within the heart: A review on the intracardiac nervous system. *J Molecular Cell Cardiology.* 2018 Jun;119:1-9.

[21] Kim HG, Cheon EJ, Bai DS, et al. Stress and Heart Rate Variability: A Meta-Analysis and Review of the Literature. *Psychiatry Investig.* 2018 Feb 28;15(3):235–245.

[22] Thayer JF, Lane RD. A model of neurovisceral integration in emotion regulation and dysregulation. *J Affective Disorders.* 2000;61(3):201-216.

[23] Baldwin GS, Brooks NJ, Robson RE, et al. DNA Double Helices Recognize Mutual Sequence Homology in a Protein Free Environment. *J Phys Chem B.* 2008 Jan 9;112(4):1060-4.

[24] Liu X, Yan X, Liu Z, et al. The Effects of Electromagnetic Fields on Human Health: Recent Advances and Future. *J Bionic Eng.* 2021 Jan 28;18:210-237.

[25] HeartMath Institute. Accessed from: https://www.heartmath.org/research/research-library/ on 12-2-2024.

[26] Mariotti A. The effects of chronic stress on health: new insights into the molecular mechanisms of brain–body communication. *Future Sci OA.* 2015 Nov 1;1(3):FSO23.

[27] Liu YZ, Wang YX, Jiang CL. Inflammation: the common pathway of stress-related diseases. *Front Hum Neurosci.* 2017;11:316.

[28] Bruce Lipton. Accessed from: https://www.brucelipton.com/think-beyond-your-genes-august-2019/ on 12-2-2024.

[29] Felitti VJ, Anda RF, Nordenberg D, et al. Relationship of Childhood Abuse and Household Dysfunction to Many of the Leading Causes of Death in Adults: The Adverse Childhood Experiences (ACE) Study. 1998 May;14(4):245-58.

[30] Oral R, Ramirez M, Coohey C, et al. Adverse childhood experiences and trauma informed care: the future of health care. *Ped Res.* 2016;79:227-33.

[31] Nelson CA, Bhutta ZA, Harris NB, et al. Adversity in childhood is linked to mental and physical health throughout life. *BMJ.* 2020 Oct 28;371:m3048.

[32] Yehuda R, Daskalakis NP, Bierer LM, et al. Holocaust Exposure Induced Intergenerational Effects on FKBP5 Methylation. *Biol Psychiatry*. 2016 Sep 1;80(5):372-80.

[33] Joseph S. Epigenetics and Intergenerational trauma. *Holistic Wellness Int Pathophysiology*. 2021 Jan.

[34] Paddison S. *The Power of the Heart*, Planetary Pub, Boulder Creek, CA, 1992.

[35] Rein G. Effect of conscious intention on human DNA> *Proc Int Forum New Sci*. 18996 Oct.

[36] Bhat US, Shahi N, Surendran S, et al. Neuropeptides and Behaviors: How Small Peptides Regulate Nervous System Function and Behavioral Outputs. *Front Mol Neurosci*. 2021 Dec 2;14:786471.

[37] Carniglia L, Ramirez D, Durand D, et al. Neuropeptides and Microglial Activation in Inflammation, Pain, and Neurodegenerative Diseases. *Mediators Inflamm*. 2017 Jan 5;2017:5048616.

[38] "Joseph Smith's Teachings about Priesthood, Temple, and Women". Accessed from: https://www.churchofjesuschrist.org/study/manual/gospel-topics-essays/joseph-smiths-teachings-about-priesthood-temple-and-women?lang=eng on 12-4-2024.

[39] Hodge DR. A Systematic Review of the Empirical Literature on Intercessory Prayer. *Res Social Work Practice*. 2007 Mar;17(2):174-87.

[40] Roberts L, Hall IAS. Intercessory prayer for the alleviation of ill health. *Cochrane Database Syst Rev*. 2007 Jan 24:(1):CD000368.

[41] Moses 3:5–7; Genesis 2:4–5.

[42] Bruce R. McConkie, *The Millennial Messiah*, 642–43

[43] Doctrine and Covenants 88:7-10, 45-47.

[44] Chen C, Niehaus JK, Dinc F, et al. Neural circuit basis of placebo pain relief. *Nature*. 2024 Jul 24;632:1092-1100.

[45] Wager TD, Atlas LY. The neuroscience of placebo effects: connecting context, learning and health. *Nat Rev Neurosci*. 2015 Jul;16(7):403-18.

[46] Hammond TC, Lin AL. Glucose Metabolism is a Better Marker for Predicting Clinical Alzheimer's Disease than Amyloid or Tau. *J Cell Immunol*. 2022;4(1):15-18.

[47] Cao F, Yang F, Li J, et al. The relationship between diabetes and the dementia risk: a meta-analysis. *Diabetology Metab Syndrome*. 2024 May 14;16(101):2024.

[48] Dai C, Tan C, Zhao L, et al. Glucose metabolism impairment in Parkinson's disease. *Brain Res Bull*. 2023 Jul:199:110672.

[49] Kaynak N, Kennel V, Rackoll T, et al. Impaired glucose metabolism and the risk of vascular events and mortality after ischemic stroke: A systematic review and meta-analysis. *Cardio Diabetology*. 2024 Aug 31;23(323):2024.

[50] Puerto-Belda V, Ruz JJ, Milla C, et al. Measuring Vibrational Modes in Living Human Cells. *PRX Life*. 2024 Jan 18;2:013003.

[51] Wohl I, Sajman J, Sherman E. Cell Surface Vibrations Distinguish Malignant from Benign Cells. *Cells*. 2023 Jul 21;12(14):1901.

[52] Rose BJ. The Vibrational Frequencies of the Human Body. Accessed from: https://www.researchgate.net/publication/354326235_The_Vibrational_Frequencies_of_the_Human_Body on 12-6-2024.

[53] NeuroLaunch. *Emotions Frequency (Hz): The Science Behind Feelings and Vibrations.* Accessed at: https://neurolaunch.com/emotions-frequency-hz/ 12-16-2024.

[54] Vallejo LJ. Stage 4 Terminal Cancer Is Miraculously Gone Day After Receiving Prayer. Accessed from: https://www.christianlearning.com/stage-4-terminal-cancer/ on 12-9-2024.

[55] NBC News. 'Miracle' Baby Who Survived 13-Hour Crash Ordeal Released From Hospital. Accessed from: https://www.nbcnews.com/nightly-news/father-says-baby-who-survived-13-hour-car-crash-ordeal-n321791 on 12-9-2024.

[56] Campione K. Baltimore Woman Clinically Dead for 45 Minutes Brought Back to Life While Daughter Gives Birth. Accessed from: https://people.com/health/baltimore-woman-clinically-dead-for-45-minutes-brought-back-to-life-while-daughter-gives-birth/ on 12-9-2024.

[57] Leidy HJ, Clifton PM, Astrup A, et al. The role of protein in weight management and disease prevention. *Am J Clin Nutr.* 2015 Jun;101(6):1320S-1329S.

[58] Young HA, Benton D. Heart-rate variability: a biomarker to study the influence of nutrition on physiological and psychological health? *Behav Pharmacol.* 2018 Mar 15;29(2-):140–151.

[59] Dai J, Lampert R, Wilson PW, et al. Mediterranean dietary pattern is associated with improved cardiac autonomic function among middle-aged men: a twin study. *Circ Cardiovasc Qual Outcomes.* 2010;3:366–373.

[60] Billman GE. The effects of omega-3 polyunsaturated fatty acids on cardiac rhythm: a critical reassessment. *Pharmacol Ther.* 2013;140:53–80.

[61] Popp FA. Properties of biophotons and their theoretical implications. *Indian J Exp Biol.* 2003 May;41(5):391-402.

[62] Ammar A, Trabelsi K, Boukhris O, et al. Effects of Polyphenol-Rich Interventions on Cognition and Brain Health in Healthy Young and Middle-Aged Adults: Systematic Review and Meta-Analysis. *J Clin Med.* 2020 May 25;9(5):1598.

[63] Gomez-Pinilla F, Nguyen TTJ. Natural mood foods: The actions of polyphenols against psychiatric and cognitive disorders. *Nutr Neurosci.* 2012 May;15(3):127-33.

[64] Sandberg JC. Bjorck IME, Nilsson AC. Increased Plasma Brain-Derived Neurotrophic Factor 10.5 h after Intake of Whole Grain Rye-Based Products in Healthy Subjects. *Nutrients.* 2018 Aug 16;10(8):1097.

[65] Suzuki T, Kojima N, Osuka Y, et al. The Effects of Mold-Fermented Cheese on Brain-Derived Neurotrophic Factor in Community-Dwelling Older Japanese Women With Mild Cognitive Impairment: A Randomized, Controlled, Crossover Trial. *J Am Med Dir Assoc.* 2019 Dec;20(12):1509-1514.e2.

[66] Rana JS, Liu JY, Sidney S, et al. Risk of atherosclerotic cardiovascular disease by cardiovascular health metric categories in approximately 1 million patients. *Eur J Prev Cardiol.* 2021 Jul 23;28(8):e29-e32.

[67] Hamburg NM, McMacklin CJ, Huang AL, et al. Physical Inactivity Rapidly Induces Insulin Resistance and Microvascular Dysfunction in Healthy Volunteers. *Arterioscler Thromb Vasc Biol.* 2007 Dec;27(12):2650-6.

[68] Codella R, Chirico A. Physical Inactivity and Depression: The Gloomy Dual with Rising Costs in a Large-Scale Emergency. *Int J Environ Res Public Health.* 2023 Jan 16;20(2):1603.

[69] Diao X, Ling Y, Zeng Y, et al. Physical activity and cancer risk: a dose-response analysis for the Global Burden of Disease Study 2019. *Cancer Commun* (Lond). 2023 Nov;43(11):1229-1243.

[70] Lin TW, Tsai SF, Kuo Y. Physical Exercise Enhances Neuroplasticity and Delays Alzheimer's Disease. *Brain Plast.* 2018 Dec 12;4(1):95–110.

[71] Van Wijk EP, Ackerman J, Van Wijk R. Effect of meditation on ultraweak photon emission from hands and forehead. *Forsch Komplementarmed Klass Naturheilkd.* 2005;12:107–12.

[72] Gizewski ER, Steiger R, Waibel M, et al. Short-term meditation training influences brain energy metabolism: A pilot study on 31P MR spectroscopy. *Brain Behav.* 2020 Dec 10;11(1):e01914.

[73] Krygier JR, Heathers JAJ, Shahrestani S, et al. Mindfulness meditation, well-being, and heart rate variability: a preliminary investigation into the impact of intensive Vipassana meditation. *Int J Psychophysiol.* 2013 Sep;89(3):305-13.

[74] Kirk U, Axelsen JL. Heart rate variability is enhanced during mindfulness practice: A randomized controlled trial involving a 10-day online-based mindfulness intervention. *PLoS One.* 2020 Dec 17;15(12):e0243488.

[75] Zaccaro A, Piarulli A, Laurino M, et al. How Breath-Control Can Change Your Life: A Systematic Review on Psycho-Physiological Correlates of Slow Breathing. *Front Hum Neurosci.* 2018 Sep 7;12:353.

[76] Jain S, Hammerschlag R, Mills P, et al. Clinical Studies of Biofield Therapies: Summary, Methodological Challenges, and Recommendations. *Glob Adv Health Med.* 2015 Nov 1;4(Suppl):58–66.

[77] Rubik B, Jabs H. Effects of intention, energy healing, and mind-body states on biophoton emission. *Cosmos History: J Nat Social Philosophy.* 2017;13(2):227-47.

[78] Liester MB. Personality changes following heart transplantation: The role of cellular memory. *Med Hypotheses.* 2020 Feb:135:109468.

[79] Hou CC, Hu YN, Kuo LP, et al. Biopsychosocial Effects of Donor Traits on Heart Transplant Recipients. *Ann Transplant.* 2024 Nov 12:29:e945828.

[80] Cleve Backster. *Primary Perception: Biocommunication with plants, living foods, and human cells.* (2003) White Rose Millennium Press.

[81] Soh KS. Bonghan duct and acupuncture meridian as optical channel of biophoton. *J Korean Phys Soc.* 2004;45:1196–8.

[82] Chung JWY, Yan VCM, Zhang H. Effect of Acupuncture on Heart Rate Variability: A Systematic Review. *Evid Based Complement Alternat Med.* 2014 Feb 12;2014:819871.

[83] Sheng-xing MA. Biophysical and Biochemical Studies of Low Electrical Resistance Properties of Acupuncture Points: Roles of NOergic Signaling Molecules and Neuropeptides in Skin Electrical Conductance. *Chin J Integr Med.* 2021 Jul 28;27(8):563–569.

[84] Li H, Yajun Y, Jun H, et al. An insight into acupoints and meridians in human body based on interstitial fluid circulation. 2020 Dec. Preprint.

[85] Li HY, Wang F, Chen M, et al. An acupoint-originated human interstitial fluid circulatory network. *Chin Med J (Engl).* 2021 Sep 21;134(19):2365–2369.

[86] Ulloa L. Electroacupuncture activates neurons to switch off inflammation. *Nature.* 2021 Oct;598(7882):573–574.

[87] Sparoow K, Golianu B. Does Acupuncture Reduce Stress Over Time? A Clinical Heart Rate Variability Study in Hypertensive Patients. *Med Acupunct.* 2014 Oct 1;26(5):286–294.

[88] Kent JB, Jin L, Li XJ. Quantifying Biofield Therapy through Biophoton Emission in a Cellular Model. *J Sci Explor.* 2020;34(3):434-54.

[89] McManus DE. Reiki Is Better Than Placebo and Has Broad Potential as a Complementary Health Therapy. *J Evid Based Complementary Altern Med.* 2017 Sep 5;22(4):1051–1057.

[90] Miles P, True G. Reiki--review of a biofield therapy history, theory, practice, and research. *Altern Ther Health Med.* 2003 Mar-Apr;9(2):62-72.

[91] Dyer NL, Baldwin AL, Rand WL. A Large-Scale Effectiveness Trial of Reiki for Physical and Psychological Health. *J Altern Complement Med.* 2019;25(12):1156-1162.

[92] Billot M, Daycard M, Wood C, et al. Reiki therapy for pain, anxiety and quality of life. *BMJ Support Palliat Care.* 2019;9(4):434-438.

[93] Thrane S, Cohen SM. Effect of Reiki therapy on pain and anxiety in adults: an in-depth literature review of randomized trials with effect size calculations. *Pain Manag Nurs.* 2014;15(4):897-908.

[94] Joyce J, Herbison GP. Reiki for depression and anxiety. *Cochrane Database Syst Rev.* 2015;(4):CD006833.

[95] Topdemir EA, Saritas S. The effect of preoperative Reiki application on patient anxiety levels. Explore (NY). 2020;S1550-8307(20)30040-9.

[96] Friedman RS, Burg MM, Miles P, et al. Effects of Reiki on autonomic activity early after acute coronary syndrome. *J Am Coll Cardiol.* 2010;56(12):995-996.

[97] Seto A, Kusaka C, Sieki N, et al. Detection of extraordinary large bio-magnetic field strength from human hand during external qi emission. *Acupuncture Electro-Ther Res.* 1992;17(2):75-94.

[98] Hisamitsu T, Seto A, Nakazato S, et al. Emission of extremely strong magnetic fields from the head and whole body during oriental breathing exercises. *Acupunct Electrother Res.* 1996 Jul-Dec;21(3-4):219-27.

[99] Kokubo H, Yamamato M, Kawano K. Standard Evaluation Method of Non-contact Healing Using Biophotons. *J Int Soc Life Info Sci.* 2007;25(1):30-39.

[100] Jian-Zhou Z, Jing-Zhen L, Qing-Nian H. Statistical brain topographic mapping analysis for EEGs recorded during Qi Gong state. *Int J Neurosci.* 1988;38(3-4):415-25.

[101] Zhang JZ,ZhaoJ,HeQN.EEG findings during special psychical state (QiGong state) by means of compressed spectral array and topographic mapping. *Comput BiolMed.* 1988;18(6):455–463.

[102] Kawano K, KoitoH, FujikiT, et al. EEG and topography during Chinese "Qigong" training. *Neurosciences.* 1990;16:503–508.

[103] Pan W, Zhang L, Xia Y. The difference in EEG theta waves between concentrative and non-concentrative qigong states--a power spectrum and topographic mapping study. *J Tradit Chin Med.* 1994 Sep;14(3):212-8.

[104] Davis T, Friesen MA, Lindgren V, et al. The Effect of Healing Touch on Critical Care Patients' Vital Signs: A Pilot Study. *Holistic Nurs Prac.* 2020 Jul/Aug;34(4):244-51.

[105] Gentile D, Boselli D, O'Neill G, et al. Cancer pain relief after healing touch and massage. *J Altern Complement Med.* 2018;24(9-10):968-973.

[106] Cook C, Guerrerio JF, Slater VE, eta l. Healing touch and quality of life in women receiving radiation treatment for cancer: a randomized controlled trial. *Altern Ther Health Med.* 2004 May-Jun;10(3):34-41.

[107] Jain S, McMahon GF, Hasen P, et al. Healing touch with guided imagery for PTSD in returning active duty military: a randomized controlled trial. *Mil Med.* 2012;177(9):1015-1021.

[108] MacIntyre B, Hamilton J, Fricke T, et al. The efficacy of healing touch in coronary artery bypass surgery recovery: a randomized clinical trial. *Altern Ther Health Med.* 2008;14(4):24-32.

[109] Brown CC, Fischer R, Wagman AMI, et al. The EEG in meditation and therapeutic touch healing. J Altered States Conscious. 1977;3(2):169-180

[110] Green EE, Parks PA, Guyer PM, et al. Anomalous electrostatic phenomena in exceptional subjects.
Subtle Energies. 1991;2(3):69-94

[111] Quinn JF, Strelkauskas AJ. Psychoimmunologic effects of therapeutic touch on practitioners and recently bereaved recipients: a pilot study. *ANS Adv Nurs Sci.* 1993;15(4):13-26.

[112] Coakley AB, Duffy ME. The effect of therapeutic touch on postoperative patients. *J Holist Nurs.* 2010;28(3):193-200.

[113] Tabatabaee A, Tafreshi MZ, Rassouli M, Aledavood SA, AlaviMajd H, Farahmand SK. Effect of therapeutic touch in patients with cancer: a literature review. *Med Arch.* 2016;70(2):142-7.

[114] Kumarappah A, Senderovich H. Therapeutic touch in the management of responsive behavior in patients with dementia. *Adv Mind Body Med.* 2016 Fall;30(4):8-13.

[115] Mueller G, Palli C, Schumacher P. The effect of therapeutic touch on back pain in adults on a neurological unit: an experimental pilot study. *Pain Manag Nurs*. 2019;20(1):75-81.

[116] Sujianto MU, Johan A. Effects of Therapeutic Touch to Reduce Anxiety As a Complementary Therapy: A Systematic Review. *KnE Life Sciences*. 2019.

[117] Belal M, Vijayakumar V, Prasad K N, et al. Perception of Subtle Energy " Prana", and Its Effects During Biofield Practices: A Qualitative Meta-Synthesis. *Glob Adv Integr Med Health*. 2023 Sep 12:12:27536130231200477.

[118] Jaisri G, Dayananda G, Saraswathi H, et al. Heart Rate Variability during meditation in Pranic Healers. *NJIRM*. 2011 Oct-Dec;2(4):113-116.

[119] Sugano H, Uchida S, Kuramoto I. A new approach to the studies of subtle energies. *Subtle Energies*. 1994;5(2):143-166.

[120] Gasiorowska A, Navarro-Rodriguez T, Dickman R, et al. Clinical trial: the effect of Johrei on symptoms of patients with functional chest pain. *Aliment Pharmacol Ther*. 2009 Jan;29(1):126-34.

[121] Becker RO, Selden G. (1985). *The body electric: Electromagnetism and the foundation of life*. William Morrow & Co.

[122] Joseph P, Acharya UR, Poo CK, et al. Effect of reflexological stimulation on heart rate variability. *ITBM-RBM*. 2004 Apr;25(1):40-45.

[123] Zhen LP, Fatimah SN, Acharya U R, et al. Study of heart rate variability due to reflexological stimulation. *Clin Acupuncture Oriental Med*. 2003 Dec;4(4):173-78.

[124] Jones J, Thomson P, Lauder W, et al. Reflexology has an acute (immediate) haemodynamic effect in healthy volunteers: a double-blind randomised controlled trial. *Complement Ther Clin Pract*. 2012 Nov;18(4):204-11.

[125] Exodus 7:9–12; Numbers 17:8.

[126] Numbers 21:5-7.

[127] 2 Kings 2:8.

[128] No author listed. *Divining Rods*. Accessed from: https://www.churchofjesuschrist.org/study/history/topics/divining-rods?lang=eng#p1 on 12-16-2024.

[129] No author listed. *Urim and Thummim*. Accessed at: https://www.churchofjesuschrist.org/study/manual/gospel-topics/urim-and-thummim?lang=eng#title1 on 12-16-2024.

[130] Ether 3:1-6.

[131] Goldsby TL, Goldsby ME, McWalters M, et al. Effects of Singing Bowl Sound Meditation on Mood, Tension, and Well-being: An Observational Study. *J Evid Based Complementary Altern Med*. 2016 Sep 30;22(3):401–406.

[132] Goldsby TL, Goldsby ME. Eastern Integrative Medicine and Ancient Sound Healing Treatments for Stress: Recent Research Advances. *Integr Med* (Encinitas). 2020 Dec;19(6):24–30.

[133] Seetharaman R, Avhad S, Rane J. Exploring the healing power of singing bowls: An overview of key findings and potential benefits. *Explore*. 2024 Jan-Feb;20(1):39-43.

[134] Karakis P, Grigorios T, Theodoros K, et al. The Effectiveness of Bioresonance Method on Human Health, *Open Epidemiology J*. 2019 Apr;8(1):1-8.

[135] Muresan D, Salcudean A, Sabau DC, et al. Bioresonance therapy may treat depression. *J Med Life*. 2021 Mar-Apr;14(2):238–242.

[136] Hamblin MR. Mechanisms and applications of the anti-inflammatory effects of photobiomodulation. *AIMS Biophys*. 2017;4(3):337-361.

[137] Hamblin MR. Mechanisms and applications of the anti-inflammatory effects of photobiomodulation. *AIMS Biophys*. 2017;4(3):337-361.

[138] Roddick CM, Wang Y, Chen FS, et al. Effects of near-infrared radiation in ambient lighting on cognitive performance, emotion, and heart rate variability. *J Environ Psych*. 2024 Dec;100:102484.

[139] Chevalier G, Mori K, Oschman JL. The effect of earthing (grounding) on human physiology.*Eur Biol Bioelectromag*. 2006 Jan 31:600-21.

[140] Ghaly M, Teplitz D. The Biologic Effects of Grounding the Human Body During Sleep as Measured by Cortisol Levels and Subjective Reporting of Sleep, Pain, and Stress. *J Alt Complement Med*. 2004;10(5):767-76.

[141] Ghaly M, Teplitz D. The biological effects of grounding the human body during sleep, as measured by cortisol levels and subjective reporting of sleep, pain and stress. *J Altern Complement Med*. 2004 10(5):767-776.

[142] Chevalier G. Changes in Pulse Rate, Respiratory Rate, Blood Oxygenation, Perfusion Index, Skin Conductance, and Their Variability Induced During and After Grounding Human Subjects for 40 Minutes. *J Altern Complement Med*. 2010;16(1):81-87.

[143] Chung YH, Chen SJ, Lee CL, et al. Relaxing Effects of Breathing Pseudotsuga menziesii and Lavandula angustifolia Essential Oils on Psychophysiological Status in Older Adults. *Int J Environ Res Public Health*. 2022 Nov 18;19(22):15251.

[144] Abrahamyan HT, Minasyan SM. [Corrective effect of aromatherapy on indices of heart rate variability in students under exam stress conditions]. *Gig Sanit*. 2016;95(6):563-8.

[145] Chang KM, Shen CW. Aromatherapy Benefits Autonomic Nervous System Regulation for Elementary School Faculty in Taiwan. *Evid Based Complement Alternat Med*. 2011 Apr 10;2011:946537.

[146] Matsumoto T, Kimura T, Hayashi T. Does Japanese Citrus Fruit Yuzu (Citrus junos Sieb. ex Tanaka) Fragrance Have Lavender-Like Therapeutic Effects That Alleviate Premenstrual Emotional Symptoms? A Single-Blind Randomized Crossover Study. *J Altern Complement Med*. 2017 Jun;23(6):461-470.

[147] Schneider R. Essential oil inhaler (AromaStick®) improves heat tolerance in the Hot Immersion Test (HIT). Results from two randomized, controlled experiments. *J Therm Biol*. 2020 Jan;87:102478.

[148] Sgoifo A, Carnevali L, Pattini E, et al. Psychobiological evidence of the stress resilience fostering properties of a cosmetic routine. *Int J Biol Stress*. 2021;24(1):53-63.

[149] Zafar S, Streeter TWJA, Inamdar SS, et al. Effect of Aromatherapy and Energy Medicine on the Human Biofield: A Pilot Study. Accessed from: https://www.academia.edu/16583274/Effect_of_Aromatherapy_and_Energy_Medicine_on_the_Human_Biofield_A_Pilot_Study on 12-11-2024.

[150] Sanchez-Vidana DI, Po KK, Fung TK, et al. Lavender essential oil ameliorates depression-like behavior and increases neurogenesis and dendritic complexity in rats. *Neurosci Lett*. 2019;701:180–192.

[151] Sanders C, Diego M, Fernandez M, et al. EEG asymmetry responses to lavender and rosemary aromas in adults and infants. *Int J Neurosci*. 2002;112(11):1305–1320.

[152] Moss M, Cook J, Wesnes K, et al. Aromas of rosemary and lavender essential oils differentially affect cognition and mood in healthy adults. *Int J Neurosci*. 2003;113(1):15–38.

[153] Fung TKH Lau BWM, Ngai SPC, et al. Therapeutic Effect and Mechanisms of Essential Oils in Mood Disorders: Interaction between the Nervous and Respiratory Systems. *Int J Mol Sci*. 2021 May 3;22(9):4844.

[154] Qneibi M, Bdir S, Maayeh C, et al. A Comprehensive Review of Essential Oils and Their Pharmacological Activities in Neurological Disorders: Exploring Neuroprotective Potential. *Nature*. 2023 Sep;49:258-289.

[155] Fung TKH, Lau BWM, Ngai SPC, et al. Therapeutic Effect and Mechanisms of Essential Oils in Mood Disorders: Interaction between the Nervous and Respiratory Systems. *Int J Mol Sci*. 2021 May 3;22(9):4844.

[156] Cho K, Kim M. Effects of aromatherapy on depression: A meta-analysis of randomized controlled trials. *General Hospital Psych*. 2023 Sep-Oct;84:215-25.

[157] Tan L, Lao FF, Long LZ, et al. Essential oils for treating anxiety: a systematic review of randomized controlled trials and network meta-analysis. *Front Public Health*. 2023 Jun 1:11:1144404.

[158] Kokburn K, Nemoto K, Yamakawa Y. Continuous inhalation of essential oil increases gray matter volume. *Brain Res Bull*. 2024;208(2024):110896.

[159] Dintica CS, Marseglia A, Rizzuto D, et al. Impaired olfaction is associated with cognitive decline and neurodegeneration in the brain. *Neurology*. 2019 Feb 12;92(7):e700–e709.

[160] Woo CC, Miranda B, Sathishkumar M, et al. Overnight olfactory enrichment using an odorant diffuser improves memory and modifies the uncinate fasciculus in older adults. *Front Neurosci*. 2023 Jul 24:17:1200448.

[161] Passarelli S, Free CM, Shepon A, et al. Global estimation of dietary micronutrient inadequacies: a modelling analysis. 2024 Oct;12(10):E1590-99.

[162] Pomportes L, Davranche K, Brisswalter I, et al. Heart rate variability and cognitive function following a multi-vitamin and mineral supplementation with added guarana (Paullinia cupana). *Nutrients*. 2014 Dec 31;7(1):196-208.

[163] Lopresti AL. Association between Micronutrients and Heart Rate Variability: A Review of Human Studies. *Adv Nutr*. 2020 May 1;11(3):559-575.

[164] Zenk F, Loeser E, Schiavo R, et al. Germ line-inherited H3K27me3 restricts enhancer function during maternal-to-zygotic transition. *Science*. 2017 Jul 14; 357(6347): 212-216.

[165] van Abeelen AF, Elias SG, Bossuyt PM, et al. Famine exposure in the young and the risk of type 2 diabetes in adulthood. *Diabetes*. 2012;61(9):2255-2260.

[166] Borge TC, Aase H, Brantsæter AL, et al. The importance of maternal diet quality during pregnancy on cognitive and behavioural outcomes in children: a systematic review and meta-analysis. *BMJ Open*. 2017;7(9):e016777.

[167] Diniz F, Edgington-Giordano F, Ngo NYN, et al. Morphometric analysis of the intergenerational effects of protein restriction on nephron endowment in mice. *Heliyon*. 2024;10(20):e39552.

[168] Jawaid A, Jehle KL, Mansuy IM. Impact of Parental Exposure on Offspring Health in Humans. *Trends Genetics*. 2021 Apr;37(4):373-88.

[169] Ornellas F, Carapeto PV, Mandarin-de Lacerda CA, et al. Obese fathers lead to an altered metabolism and obesity in their children in adulthood: review of experimental and human studies. *J Pediatrics*. 2017 Nov-Dec;93(6):551-9.

[170] Bhadsavle SS, Golding MC. Paternal epigenetic influences on placental health and their impacts on offspring development and disease. *Front Genet*. 2022 Nov 18;13:1068408.

[171] Sucharita S, Dwarkanath P, Thomas T, et al. Low maternal vitamin B12 status during pregnancy is associated with reduced heart rate variability indices in young children. *Matern Child Nutr*. 2012 May 24;10(2):226–233.

[172] Solati Z, Jazayeri S, Tehrani-Doost M, et al. Zinc monotherapy increases serum brain-derived neurotrophic factor (BDNF) levels and decreases depressive symptoms in overweight or obese subjects: a double-blind, randomized, placebo-controlled trial. *Nutr Neurosci*. 2015 May;18(4):162-8.

[173] Yu JJ, Pei LB, Zhang Y, et al. Chronic Supplementation of Curcumin Enhances the Efficacy of Antidepressants in Major Depressive Disorder: A Randomized, Double-Blind, Placebo-Controlled Pilot Study. *J Clin Psychopharmacol*. 2015 Aug;35(4):406-10.

[174] Kim CS, Cha L, Sim M, et al. Probiotic Supplementation Improves Cognitive Function and Mood with Changes in Gut Microbiota in Community-Dwelling Older Adults: A Randomized, Double-Blind, Placebo-Controlled, Multicenter Trial. *J Gerontol A Biol Sci Med Sci*. 2021 Jan 1;76(1):32-40.

[175] Haghighat N, Rajabi S, Mohammashahi M. Effect of synbiotic and probiotic supplementation on serum brain-derived neurotrophic factor level, depression and anxiety symptoms in hemodialysis patients: a randomized, double-blinded, clinical trial. *Nutr Neurosci*. 2021 Jun;24(6):490-499.

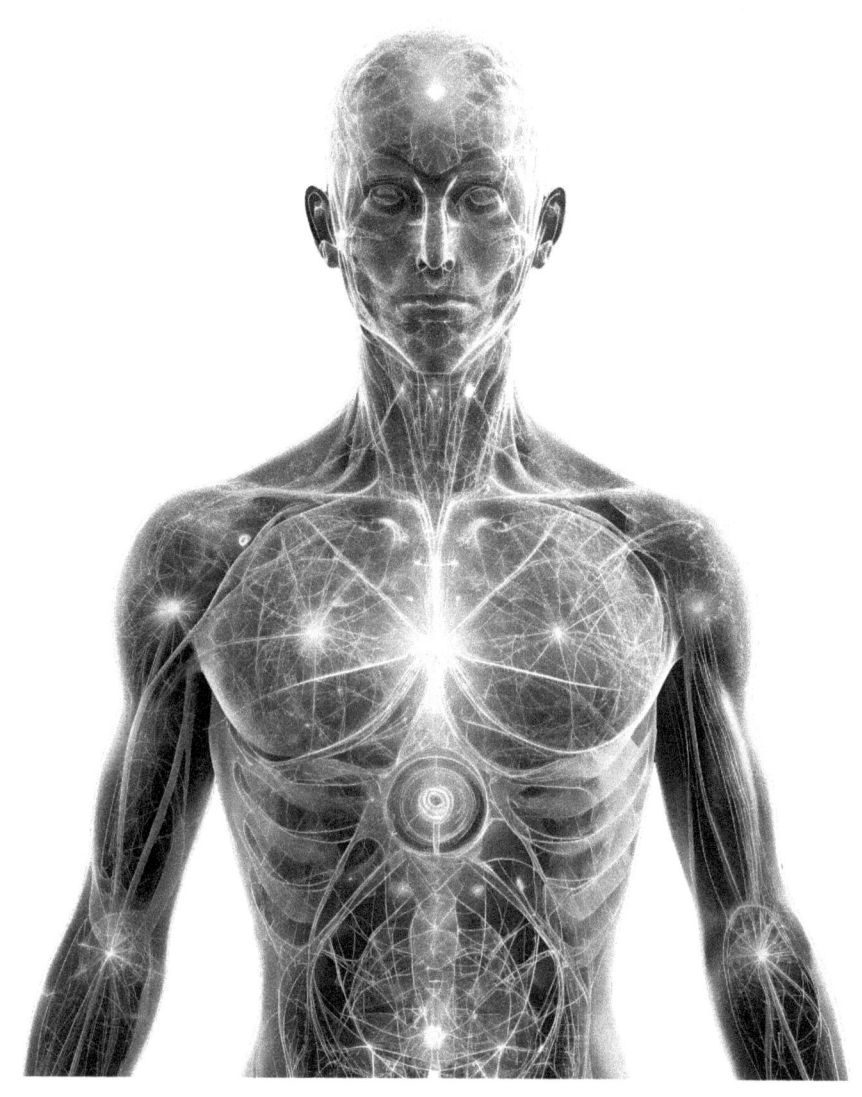

Index

A
acupressure, 100, 109-111, 132
acupuncture, 17, 100, 109-112, 139, 148
ATP, 14, 72, 87, 96, 149, 151

B
BDNF, 72, 86, 90-91, 94, 170-172
belief, VII, VIII, 12, 19, 20, 34, 57, 58, 59, 60, 62, 63, 67, 70, 71, 79, 83, 84, 85, 100, 120, 128, 129, 137, 138, 180
binaural beats, 142, 143
biochemical, 11, 15, 27, 45, 51, 52, 68, 92
bioelectrical, 11, 13, 76, 108
bioenergetics, 12, 14, 17, 21, 22, 31
biofeedback, 147, 158
biofield, 22-24, 42, 69, 86, 93-94, 99-103, 108, 110, 111, 113, 114, 115, 118, 121, 128, 132, 143, 144, 145, 150, 153, 155, 162-163, 165, 175, 176, 178, 183
biophotons, 8, 17, 60-64, 65, 69, 86, 89, 92-93, 95, 103, 109, 113, 115, 118, 119, 145, 147-148, 149, 152, 165, 175, 176, 183
bioresonance, 141, 144-147, 158
bioresonance therapy, 141, 144-147
body memory, 104, 106
brainwaves, 29, 69, 76, 119, 124, 127, 143, 160

C
cellular memory, 24, 33, 42-44, 45, 85, 92, 104, 107
Chiren 3.0, 148
Christ, Jesus, 53, 55-56, 59, 60, 85, 175, 176, 181, 182
Christianity, 57-60, 138
coherence, 23, 33-35, 37, 45, 62, 69, 76, 85, 95-97, 109, 110, 111, 112, 113, 116, 143, 144, 150, 154, 155, 158, 161, 165, 168
consciousness and intention, 62-63
cortisol, 23, 39-40, 41, 105, 106, 112, 113, 125, 156-157, 162, 171
crystals, 101, 137-138, 143

D
DNA, 24, 26-29, 41, 43-44, 93, 102, 170

E
earthing, 154-157
Einstein, Albert, 11-12, 30
electrical impedance tomography, 16, 18
electrocardiography, 16, 115, 123,
electroencephalography, 16, 73, 118, 119, 124, 130, 131, 156
electromyography, 16, 156
emotional transference, 121-122
energetic resonance, 63, 132
energy transfer, 103
entrainment, 66
epigenetics, 41-42, 44, 106, 107, 169
essential oils, 18, 47, 159-166, 177, 179

F
faith, VII-IX, 52, 55-57, 59, 65, 69-71, 77, 79, 80, 138, 175, 177, 180, 181-182, 183
foot zoning, 140

frequency, 12, 22, 29, 35-36, 61, 63, 66, 69, 74-77, 86, 88, 89, 97, 111, 112, 113, 115, 129, 133, 137, 142, 143, 145, 150, 153, 154, 160, 161, 162, 165, 170, 178

G

genetically modified organisms (GMOs), 90
God, VII-IX, 24, 52, 53, 55, 56, 57, 59, 60, 61, 62, 64, 77, 79, 80, 84, 85, 99, 138, 139, 166, 172, 175, 176, 181
grounding, 154-157

H

healing touch, 100, 119-124, 177
health span, 92, 168
heart rate variability, 18, 22, 25, 26, 34, 35, 37, 86, 88, 89, 96-97, 102, 110, 111, 115, 129, 133-134, 143, 145, 150, 152, 153, 155, 157, 159, 160, 161, 168-169, 170, 175, 176, 180, 183
HeartMath Institute, 33, 34, 37, 42
herbs, 18, 99, 166-177
Holy Spirit, 56
hope, 55, 69-71, 123, 181
HPAA, 38, 40, 41, 50

I

immune surveillance, 49-50
intrinsic cardiac nervous system, 25-26

J

Jesus Christ, 53, 55-56, 59, 60, 85, 175, 176, 181, 182
Johrei, 100, 129-131

K

kinesiology, 17, 100, 131-132

L

light therapy, 141, 148-154, 158, 177, 178, 183
limbic system, 24
low-level laser therapy, 149

M

magnetic field, 16, 17, 21, 23, 29, 30, 34, 117-120, 145
magnetoencephalography, 16
massage, 100, 119-124,
meditation, 11, 61, 63, 70, 73, 74, 95-97, 100, 116, 124, 129, 130, 136, 143, 178, 179, 180
micronutrients, 167, 168, 169
microRNA, 106-107
mindfulness, 45, 70, 74, 95-97, 116, 133, 177
mRNA, 72
MTHFR, 169-170

N

neural highway, 98
neuroplasticity, 26, 69, 71-74, 86, 90, 94, 170, 171, 175
neuroscience, 98
neurotransmitter, 19, 26, 54, 93, 105, 106, 112, 163
nocebo effect,
nutrigenomics, 87-88
nutrition, 14, 18, 47, 48, 51, 61, 77, 85, 86-91, 97, 108, 167, 171, 177, 179

P

parasympathetic nervous system, 35-37, 115, 129, 155, 157, 161
photobiomodulation, 18, 149, 151, 178
physical activity, 88, 92-95, 97
physics, 12-13, 14, 17, 57, 61, 76, 144
placebo effect, 19-21, 71, 73, 101, 113, 126, 138, 157, 162, 168, 171, 172
pranic healing, 100, 127-129
prayer, VIII, 11, 45, 55, 56-57, 59, 60, 63, 65, 70, 73, 74, 77, 85, 101, 118, 135, 136,
probiotics, 171, 172
pulsed electromagnetic fields, 32
pulsed electromagnetic field (PEMF) therapy, 21

Q

qigong, 17, 22, 100, 116-119
quantum biology, 12, 14-15, 28, 31, 108
quantum entanglement, 63-64, 104

R

radiant energy, 32
red-light therapy, 149, 151-154
reflexology, 100, 133-135, 174, 184
Reiki, 17, 100, 112-116, 139, 177

S

sacred geometry, 62
scientism, 79
self-healing, 47-50, 144, 147, 148
sound therapy, 141, 142-144, 183
sound waves, 66

spirituality, 57, 65, 74, 116, 136, 138, 158, 159, 181
sympathetic nervous system, 35, 157, 170

T

Tesla Coils, 32
Tesla, Nikola, 12, 30, 32
The Healing Code, 101, 135-136
therapeutic touch, 22, 100, 119-127
Tibetan singing bowl, 142-143
toxins, 47, 49, 50, 93, 169
transcutaneous electrical nerve stimulation (TENS), 21
truth declarations, 84-85, 181

V

vagus nerve, 98
vibration, 12, 61, 63, 69, 74, 75, 76, 77, 86, 89, 110, 111, 112, 113, 119, 128, 133, 137, 141, 142, 143, 144, 145, 150, 158, 162, 165, 176, 177, 178, 179,
vibrational foods, 89
violet ray devices, 32

www.ingramcontent.com/pod-product-compliance
Lightning Source LLC
Chambersburg PA
CBHW050904160426
43194CB00011B/2282